ACUPUNCTURE
FOR THE EYES

ACUPUNCTURE
FOR THE EYES

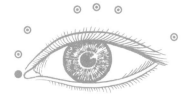

Julian Scott

EASTLAND PRESS • SEATTLE

Disclaimer

The information in this book is given in good faith and is intended to be used by qualified acupuncture practitioners only. Those who have not had a minimum of three years of training in acupuncture are strongly advised not to use this book, except under supervision.

Published by Eastland Press, Inc.
P.O. Box 99749
Seattle, WA 98139 USA
www.eastlandpress.com

International Standard Book Number: 0-939616-46-7
Library of Congress Control Number: 2005923287
Printed in the United States of America

2   4   6   8   10   9   7   5   3   1

Book design by Gary Niemeier

Table of Contents

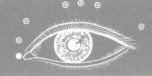

List of Illustrations

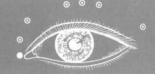

Acknowledgments

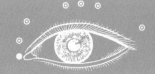

THE FIRST PERSON to show me that eye disorders could respond to natural means was Miss Olive Scarlet, a Bates' teacher who had been taught by Bates himself and who was then in her eighties. I am immensely grateful to her for starting me on the way. I would like to thank NFKA (Norwegian Society for Classical Acupuncture) for inviting me to give a talk on eye disorders. This provided the impetus for organizing my thoughts and putting them down on paper. I would like to thank Lou Radford for reading the book and making many helpful comments and Louis Poncz for editing, and during the editing, for making many helpful contributions. Finally, I would like to thank my teacher Dr. Zhang Cai-Yun for her great kindness in showing me the possibilities of acupuncture in general and in eye disorders in particular.

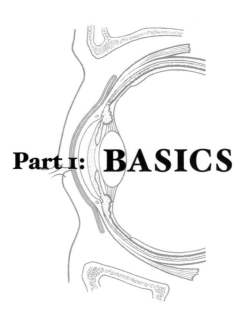

Part I: BASICS

Introduction

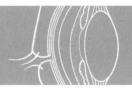

T HIS BOOK IS an introduction to the treatment of eye diseases by acupuncture. It has been written to encourage more acupuncturists to treat eye conditions. All the eye diseases in this book respond to acupuncture. In some cases this may come as a surprise. For example, it may be thought that the only way of treating a problem like corneal opacity would be the use of eye drops or an eye wash. This turns out not to be the case. Acupuncture can be extraordinarily effective in treating a wide range of conditions.

Many eye conditions are described here. At the most basic level, there are treatments to prepare patients for surgery and to help them recover afterward. These treatments should be known by all acupuncturists. At the other end, there are treatments for acute conditions that should only be attempted by experienced practitioners.

In the eye department at a TCM hospital, it is more common to have an herbalist giving treatment. However, this is largely a result of the ready availability of herbalists and the traditional hierarchy that places herbalists above acupuncturists. Most of the eye diseases that can be cured by Chinese herbs can also be cured by acupuncture, and the diseases that are difficult to cure with herbs are also difficult to cure with acupuncture. There are, however, some diseases for which acupuncture is the treatment of choice.

Sources

The information contained in this book comes mainly from Chinese texts, but this is supplemented by my own experience. Information on the use of acupuncture for eye diseases is surprisingly hard to come by. Each acupuncture book will yield a few nuggets of information, and many books must be consulted to assemble a reasonably broad range of conditions. A list of those books is provided in the bibliography.

When is acupuncture appropriate?

Acupuncture is appropriate in the treatment of many eye problems. For some conditions, such as macular degeneration and retinitis pigmentosa, which have no treatment in Western medicine, acupuncture is the treatment of choice. For other diseases, such as cataract (in the early stages) and chronic (open-angle) glaucoma, there is a treatment in orthodox medicine. However, for many patients, acupuncture may be the preferred treatment. Acupuncture can certainly be beneficial as an adjunct therapy in these conditions.

There is a third category, such as acute conjunctivitis and acute (closed-angle) glaucoma, where the disease is violent and the risks of going blind are very high. For these diseases, acupuncture can indeed offer a rapid cure — often quicker and more reliably than Western medicine — but the treatment should nevertheless be carried out in the emergency room of a hospital.

Throughout this book an attempt has been made to provide some information about the conventional treatment and how it compares with acupuncture. In any particular patient, the decision to treat with acupuncture or conventional medicine, or both, should be made carefully.

A note about the word 'cure'

From time to time, I use the word 'cure' with reference to eye problems. This is a word that has fallen out of use, and some associations of alternative practitioners forbid their members to use the word, preferring the term 'treat' or 'successfully treat.' On the whole, this is good advice when presenting the benefits of acupuncture to the public. No one can guarantee a cure. In the words of a once celebrated physician, "Every intervention is something of an experiment." To offer the certainty of a cure will certainly lead to disappointment in some patients.

Bearing this in mind, the word cure is nonetheless useful. I use it to mean changing the patient's condition so that both the symptoms and the underlying condition disappear. With this type of change, it is unlikely that the illness or the symptoms will return. I distinguish between curing a condition and supporting a patient. In many of the conditions covered here, a complete cure is unlikely, but the body may be supported sufficiently to remove all unpleasant symptoms. I would consider this to be 'effectively treated.'

Results of treatment

Throughout the text, I have tried to provide some idea of the effectiveness of acupuncture treatment. For some conditions, this is based on my own experience, and for others, it is based on Chinese sources. These sources require some comment since the results are usually presented in the form, "x patients were cured, y patients had partial improvement, and z patients had no improvement." This sort of clinical result is far from scientific. It seems to be based on the opinion of the practitioner, and, from my own personal experience, I know how unreliable that can be. The results, however, should not be dismissed. Unscientific they may be, but they are nevertheless significant because they provide at least an impression of the results that can be obtained.

Chapter 1

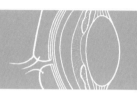

Anatomy and Physiology

1.1 Structure of the Eye

The structure of the eye is complicated. Fortunately, however, as acupuncturists we do not need to know the structure in great detail. Yet some knowledge of the structure and function of the eye, beyond what can be inferred merely by looking at it from the outside, is useful in understanding the treatment of its many conditions. We will begin at the front of the eye (Fig. 1.1).

Cornea

The cornea is in the very front part, and consists of a clear meniscus that allows light to pass into the eye. It is called the 'cornea' because it is horny and hard (*cornus* is Latin for 'horn'). In some ways, the material is similar to that of a fingernail, but there is a difference—the cornea is made of living tissue. It has many nerves, which is what makes it so sensitive to touch and to foreign bodies, and it is awash in lymphatic fluid, which nourishes the tissue. Accordingly, the cornea is somewhat akin to hard skin, and this provides a clue to the diseases to which it is prone, for example, corneal ulcer and corneal erosion, which are similar to ulcers and eczema in their underlying imbalance. The cornea can also become opaque when its layers of tissue become waterlogged.

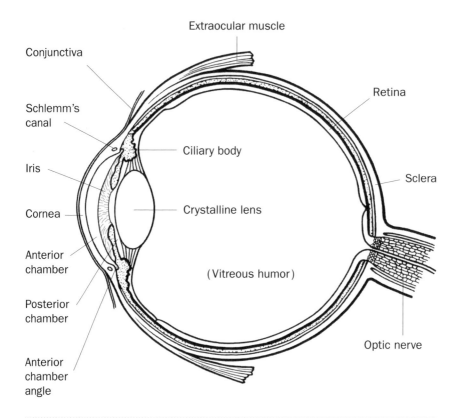

Fig. 1.1 Anatomy of the eye

Aqueous humor

This fluid, which is called 'aqueous' because it has the same refractive index as water, fills the cavity between the cornea and the lens. The fluid is constantly flowing. It is secreted by the choroid and drains out through a network of tiny capillaries that collect into Schlemm's canal, which is located in the ciliary body.

Conjunctiva

This thin, transparent membrane covers the front of the sclera and the inside part of the eyelids. It is the 'skin' that protects the eye from external factors. As a result, it is easily injured or infected.

Inner and outer canthus

The inner canthus is the small red area at the angle formed by the medial meeting point of the upper and lower eyelids. The outer canthus is the angle formed at the lateral meeting point of the eyelids.

Sclera

The sclera (Σκλερος is Greek for 'hard') is the 'white' of the eye. It is the sclera that makes up most of the structure of the eye—the rest of the globe. As its name suggests, it is extremely tough, which is of importance to acupuncture practitioners since many people are afraid of needling points like ST-1 *(cheng qi)* to any depth for fear of injuring the sclera. The sclera is in fact so tough that it would be almost impossible to puncture it with a normal acupuncture needle. It would be possible to scratch it, however, which would be painful for it is richly endowed with nerves.

Iris

This diaphragm gives the eye its characteristic color. Its function is to control the amount of light that enters the eye. In bright light, the iris contracts, leaving just a pinhole for the light to get through, while in low light, it enlarges, allowing more light to get through. The iris is quite thin, and it needs the support of the lens behind it. In people who have had the lens removed, the iris can be seen waving around like seaweed on the ocean floor. The iris is contracted by a sphincter muscle that goes all around the inner part, and it is dilated by a sheet of muscle that covers the whole of the posterior side.

Lens

The lens needs little explanation. It was the envy of optical engineers because its surfaces are not spherical. Only recently has it been possible to design and make nonspherical lenses from glass. Unlike the cornea, the lens is more or less dead. It does not constantly renew itself, or at least it does so only very slowly. Consequently, as time goes on, it takes on the characteristics that you would expect from any clear plastic—it gradually becomes less flexible and slightly opaque. This is the reason why focusing becomes more difficult and cataracts (opacity) appear as age creeps on.

Ciliary body

This muscle, which is covered by many folds, focuses the lens. Unlike most muscles, it becomes *longer* as it contracts so that it pushes the lens inward. This makes the lens fatter, thereby reducing its focal length. Because of this muscle, objects that are nearby can be brought into focus. The ciliary body also has the function of secreting the aqueous humor.

Vitreous humor

This is a clear, gelatinous substance that fills the space behind the lens. It is attached to the inner surface of the eye. It is permeated by the same fluid that forms the aqueous humor. It is called 'vitreous' because it has the same refractive index as glass.

Retina

This network of nerve cells (ρετινα is Greek for 'net') at the back of the eye converts light into nerve impulses. The retina is anatomically an extension of the brain, and it has been shown that some basic image processing takes place here before nerve impulses are transmitted to the brain proper. Strictly speaking, the retina consists merely of nerve cells and as such is not sensitive to light. The tissue becomes sensitive when it is bathed in *visual purple*.[1] When light shines on it, the visual purple becomes bleached, and in the process, chemicals are emitted that stimulate the nerves of the retina. This has clinical significance, for the supply of visual purple can go wrong, leading to the pathological condition known as retinitis pigmentosa where the pigment cells that generate the visual purple coagulate into clumps, rather than uniformly cover the whole of the retina. Over time, this gradually leads to blindness.

The retina is divided into an inner disc, known as the macula, which has higher resolution and is more sensitive to color; and an outer part, known just as the retina, which has lower spatial resolution but is more sensitive to light and much more sensitive to movement. Hence, faint stars that cannot be seen in the central field of vision can sometimes be seen in the peripheral field. Likewise, slight movements and flickers are easily detected 'out of the corner of the eye.' Finally, the retina is nourished by a network of blood vessels called the choroid, which can be clearly seen when examining the eye.

Trabecula and Schlemm's canal

These microscopic structures are located at the boundary of the cornea and the iris, just anterior to the iris. Schlemm's canal is a tiny drainage canal through which fluids drain out of the eye. The trabecula is a sieve-like network of capillaries connecting Schlemm's canal to the aqueous humor; as such, it is the portal through which fluids reach the canal. These two structures can play an important role in the development of glaucoma because the iris can fold over and block the flow of fluid into the trabecula, resulting in an increase in pressure in the eye.

1.2   Fluids of the Eye

Internal

The aqueous humor is thought to be secreted by a part of the ciliary body (Fig. 1.2). The aqueous humor diffuses out of the eye via Schlemm's canal into the blood.

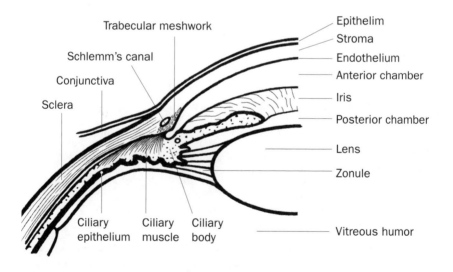

Fig. 1.2   Details of the structure of the front of the eye, showing the iris, the ciliary body, and fluid circulation

External

Tears are produced by lachrymal ducts and are part of the fluids that lubricate the movement of the eye and the eyelid. They are stabilized by a thin film of a lipid called the meibonium, which is secreted by tiny glands in the eyelids. This oily film prevents the rapid evaporation of the tears. When there is insufficient secretion, the lubricating tear film breaks up and dries out, leading to dry and irritated eyes.

Underneath the wet tear film, next to the conjunctiva, there is a thin film of mucus. As is traditional in Chinese Medicine, this thin film of mucus is said to be connected to the Lungs since it is secreted by an external mucosal membrane, the conjunctiva.

1.3   Innervation and the Extraocular Muscles

Optic nerve

This nerve carries the nervous impulse from the retina to the brain. In glaucoma, it can be damaged in the course of being pushed out by excessively high pressure in the eye. It can also be damaged by growths in the area, for example, an enlarged pituitary.

Cranial nerves

By a quirk of evolution, the muscles at the front of the eye are controlled by the cranial nerves, as shown in the following chart:

Cranial nerve	Controls
3rd	Contraction of the iris, lateral, inferior, medial rectus, and inferior oblique muscles
4th	Superior oblique muscle
5th	Cornea
6th	Lateral rectus
7th	Eyelids

These nerves come out of the cranium near GB-20 *(feng chi),* which may explains its effectiveness in treating many eye disorders.

Extraocular muscles

These muscles are used primarily for altering the direction of the eye. They consist of the inferior, superior, lateral, and medial rectus, and the inferior and superior oblique muscles (Fig. 1.3).

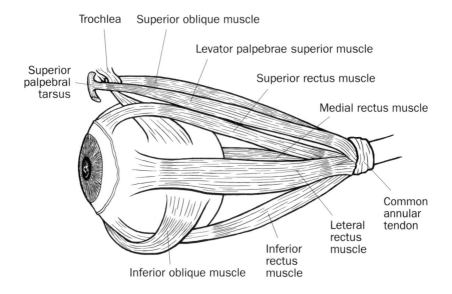

Fig. 1.3   Extraocular muscles

Endnote

1. Visual purple is the common name for rhodopsin, a chromoprotein (a protein linked to a pigment). Vitamin A is necessary for its production, hence the importance of vitamin A for healthy eyesight.

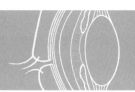

Chapter 2

The Organs and the Eyes

"The Liver opens into the eyes" is the phrase learned in the first year of training in Chinese medicine, and for many practitioners, their interest in eye problems stops there. For others, it may mean that the point LR-3 *(tai chong)* is used for treating all eye problems. This approach, however, is much too simplistic, and in practice, all the organs have some relation to the eyes.

In this section we will look at each yin organ and see how it affects the eye. First, the traditional relationship between the organ and the eye is described. Then the more recent understanding of the relationship will be provided.

2.1   Traditional View

The traditional view, found, for example, in the *Inner Classic (Nei jing)*, is based on a simple five-phase attribution of the parts of the eye on the basis of color, as set forth in the following chart:

Organ	Color	Part of eye
Kidneys	Black	Pupil
Liver	Green/brown	Iris
Heart	Red	Inner canthus
Spleen	Yellow	Eyelids
Lung	White	Sclera

This may seem a rather simplistic summary of such a complex organ as the eye; but like so many apparently simple sayings in Chinese medicine, great truths are concealed therein. Quite apart from the possibilities that these associations suggest for the treatment of the eye, there is the very fact that *parts* of the eye are themselves associated with the internal organs. This is a conceptual leap that has not yet been made in Western ophthalmology. The specialist-focused nature of Western medicine means that the overall condition of the body is often ignored.

2.2   Later Developments

As traditional Chinese medicine expanded beyond the confines of a purely five-phase approach into a deeper understanding based on the function of the organs, so a more detailed understanding of the relationship between the organs and the eyes developed. It will be seen that the earlier, simpler approach set forth in the *Inner Classic* provided a good foundation, but it needed to be amplified. Where appropriate, the role of emotions in eye disorders is also discussed.

Liver

The Liver, which "opens into the eyes," is the primary organ relating to the eyes. It is particularly concerned with the perception of light. That is, light is perceived as light rather than just a sensation because of the Liver. Using our knowledge of Western physiology, we could say that the visual purple — chromoprotein that directly interacts with light — is governed by the Liver. In particular, we see the following Liver patterns which give rise to eye symptoms:

Disorder	Resulting eye condition
Liver blood insufficiency	Can lead to poor color discrimination; also black spots in front of the eyes*
Liver heat	Causes the various problems associated with heat affecting the eye such as conjunctivitis, glaucoma, or optic atrophy
Liver and Kidney weakness†	Opens the way for many eye diseases such as optic atrophy and related degenerative conditions, watering eyes, blocked tear duct, and glaucoma

* Note that in some schools it is taught that 'floaters,' spots or hair-shaped objects that appear to float before the eye, are a symptom of Liver blood insufficiency. It is my opinion that these are simply caused by a lack of qi in the eye. In contrast, blood insufficiency gives rise to black dots, or temporarily blind areas, such as are sometime seen in migraines.   † See next page.

Rage

There is a common expression, "blinded by rage." Of all the emotions, the uprising of rage is likely to injure the eyes.

Heart

Traditionally, the Heart does not have much to do with the eyes. On the other hand, "the Heart rules the blood vessels," and eye function is very dependent on an adequate blood supply. Because of the insight provided by Western medicine, we have a better grasp of the extent of this relationship. In particular, blood clots, hardening of the arteries, and poor blood supply can all be seen in eye pathologies, and in the past three centuries, practitioners of traditional Chinese medicine have come to recognize the connection between various Heart patterns and problems with the eyes, as shown in the following table:

Poor circulation of blood in the eyes	Seen in Heart yang deficiency (xū) conditions. It is very common in the elderly and can be the root cause of degenerative diseases such as optic nerve atrophy and macular degeneration
Blood stagnation	Found in, for example, high blood pressure and may give rise to symptoms such as retinal degeneration or intraocular bleeding

Poor circulation of blood in the eyes

Found in Heart yang deficiency conditions. Very common in the elderly, and can be the root cause of degenerative diseases such as optic nerve atrophy and macular degeneration.

Blood stasis

Found, for example, in high blood pressure. May give rise to such symptoms as retinal degeneration or intraocular bleeding.

Perception

Perception—the recognition of objects 'out there' in the material world—

---

† The Liver and Kidneys become weak in the elderly. In addition, they can also become exhausted as a result of, for example, chronic illness or a severe acute illness.

depends on the Heart. Perception is the cognitive aspect of the spirit *(shén)*, which is housed in the Heart and which interprets the visual image formed on the retina in terms of familiar objects.

"The spirit shows in the eyes"

In Chinese medicine, it is said that the spirit "shows in the eyes" and is "housed in the Heart." These sayings are of significance in the treatment of eye pathology because they indicate a very direct relationship between thinking and eye function. The attitude of a person has a direct and immediate effect on the qi in the eyes. "You could see his eyes brighten when I talked about..." and "My eyes stood out on stalks" are common expressions in Britain and are graphic descriptions of what happens to the qi in the eyes when great interest is aroused. Likewise, everyone has had the experience of the eyes 'glazing over,' that particular dullness of the eyes when the qi leaves them due to boredom. These two images graphically demonstrate how mere thought can have a strong influence on the qi of the eyes. It is this relationship that makes many chronic eye diseases so intractable.

Spleen

"The Spleen controls the flesh"; as such, the Spleen governs the fleshy parts of the eye, that is, the eyelids. In some books it is said that the upper eyelid pertains to the Spleen, which brings essence *(jīng)*, while the lower eyelid pertains to the Stomach, which separates the clear from the turbid. In yet other books it is said that the upper eyelid relates to the Lungs, and the lower eyelid to the Spleen.

The Spleen also governs the transformation and transportation of fluids. This has perhaps an even greater importance for the eye, for there are fluids both inside and outside the eye.

Fluids outside the eye

When there is fluid imbalance as a result of a Spleen disharmony, the patient may exhibit:

- Dry eyes as a result of dampness or phlegm obstructing the flow of fluids to the eyes. One way of understanding this is to visualize that the tears, which should be lubricating the eyes, are too viscous to flow.
- Excessive production of tears as a result of dampness rising up to the eyes.

- 'Bags' may appear underneath the eyes as a result of dampness collecting in the eyelids, which relate to the Spleen.[1]

FLUIDS INSIDE THE EYE

The fluid that makes up the aqueous humor in the eye is continuously flowing. If the fluids in the body become too thick and viscous, then the aqueous humor also can become 'sticky' rather than watery, affecting its rate of flow. This is a significant cause of chronic (open-angle) glaucoma. The fluids may become thick when dampness that is present for a long time has been transformed into phlegm.

Surprisingly, this condition has not found its way into the TCM books on eye diseases. This may be because it is more of a Western problem than a Chinese problem. Perhaps this is because of the cold, phlegm-producing diet that is common in the West and because of the overall lack of exercise that is endemic in the West. This condition, where cold and thick phlegm alter the balance of fluids in the eye, is one of the few conditions where cold, rather than heat, affects the eye.

Lungs

The Lungs too have a relationship with the fluids. The Lungs are responsible for dispersing body fluids (and protective qi) all over the body to the space between the skin and muscles. And, more important to the discussion here, the Lungs govern fluid circulation in the head, especially the release of tears. Above all, tears result from sadness and grief, emotions that are closely related to the Lungs and the metal phase. In particular, the following symptoms may appear as a result of an impairment of the Lungs:

- dry eyes from Lung yin deficiency
- excessive tears from Lung qi deficiency
- excessive tears from long-term sadness
- excessive tears when wind-cold invades the Lungs

The latter include many other conditions related to either the Lungs or to the protective qi *(wèi qì)*. The Lungs also affect the circulation of fluid *inside* the eye; thus, chronic open-angle glaucoma can result from a Lung disharmony.

The other parts of the eye that are particularly related to the Lungs are the sclera and the cornea. Both of these are on the outside and are exposed to the elements. They must accommodate wind as well as variations in temperature and humidity. They are well innervated in much the same way as the skin and lungs. In particular, the following conditions may be related to the Lungs:

- conjunctivitis
- tear production when moving from a hot environment to a cold one
- corneal erosion and corneal ulcer,[2] both of which can result from Lung yin deficiency

GRIEF

Grief and sadness relate to the Lungs, and both have a strong effect on the eyes. We have seen how they can lead to excessive tear production. Equally important is the wistful longing seen in the elderly who have lost their partner. Rather than 'looking forward,' they feel that there is little left for them, and much of their time is spent 'looking back' over their lives, remembering the happy times. The effect this has on the qi can be disastrous for the eyes because when you 'look back' with the mind, the qi goes to the back of the eyes, rather than to the front; or even worse, the qi leaves the eyes altogether. It is this attitude that is behind many cases of degenerative eye disease.

Kidneys

Last, but not least, come the Kidneys, which are as important as the Liver to the overall health of the eyes. In particular, the retina, the optic nerve, the aqueous humor, the lens, and the yin of the eye in general are related to the Kidneys.

THE RETINA AND OPTIC NERVE

Both are anatomically part of the brain and are therefore governed by the Kidneys. As will be discussed in Chapter 7, the degenerative diseases that come under the general heading of optic atrophy are a result of Liver and Kidney weakness or Spleen and Kidney yang deficiency, showing the close relationship between the Kidneys and the nervous system of the eye. In addition, the conditions classified in TCM as optic atrophy are similar to other atrophy disorders (wěi bìng).[3]

THE AQUEOUS HUMOR

When the Kidneys are deficient, it is easy for fluid imbalances to occur in the eyes. In particular, open-angle glaucoma, where the pressure in the eye increases, may result from Kidney deficiency in much the same way that increases in blood pressure are often a result of Kidney yin deficiency.

THE LENS

The lens, the 'black' part of the eye, could be said to be governed by the Kidneys. This is evident in the following disorders:

- far-sightedness in old age (presbyopia), which is a result of a progressive hardening of the crystalline lens
- cataracts, which frequently result from Kidney yin deficiency

"THE KIDNEYS GOVERN OPENING AND CLOSING"

There are some conditions wherein the eyes either cannot open or cannot shut. One of these occurs after a great shock or fright, and this is because the Kidneys have been injured. The traditional explanation is that the Kidney energy is blocked by the terror and causes the eyes to stay open or shut.

2.3   Channels Going to the Eyes

The following channels go to the eyes (Fig. 2.1, see next page), a matter of special significance for acupuncturists.

Endnotes

1. In Western medicine, very large bags under the eyes are a symptom of Bright's disease, a form of nonsuppurative nephritis with albuminuria and edema. In our experience, this condition is a result of a combination of Kidney and Spleen yang deficiency. Alternatively, the condition can arise if the Kidneys' function of excretion is blocked by an accumulation of phlegm, which originally arose from a Spleen dysfunction.

2. As noted in Chapter 1, the cornea is somewhat akin to hard skin, and corneal disorders are somewhat akin to skin diseases.

3. For a more complete discussion of the atrophy disorder, see, for example, *The Practice of Chinese Medicine* (pp. 685-699) where it is referred to as *wei* disorder.

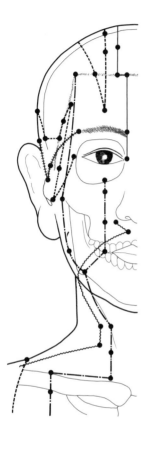

~~~~~~~~~~~ Large Intestine channel

– · – · – · Stomach channel

——————— Bladder channel

++++++++++++ Triple Burner *(san jiao)* channel

– – – – – – – Gallbladder channel

Not shown:

- The Liver channel ascends into the nasopharynx and connects with the tissues surrounding the eye.

- A branch of the Penetrating vessel *(chong mai)* curves around the lips and terminates below the eye in the nasal cavity.

- The Yang Heel vessel *(yang qiao mai)* passes beside the mouth before reaching the inner canthus of the eye, meeting the Bladder channel at BL-1 *(jing ming)* and the Stomach channel at ST-1 *(cheng qi)*, S-3 *(ju liao)*, and S-4 *(di cang)*.

- The Yin Heel vessel *(yin qiao mai)* traverses the cheek before reaching the inner canthus where it joins with the Yang Heel vessel and Bladder channel at BL-1 *(jing ming)*.

Fig. 2.1 Channels going to the eye

Chapter 3

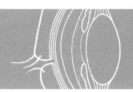

Some Diagnostic Features

Specific symptoms associated with the eyes, and their underlying TCM etiology, are shown in the following table.

Symptom	Disorder
• SENSATIONS IN THE EYE:	
Strong pain	Excess condition, usually excess heat
Itching	Deficiency condition, allowing wind to enter, or Liver heat
Extremely itchy eyes	Excess heat in the Liver channel
Dull pain in the eyes	Deficiency condition, often with cold
Continuous, stabbing pain	Blood stagnation
Intermittent stabbing pain, like a needle	Blood stagnation from qi and blood insufficiency
Eye socket and eyebrow bone pain (i.e., sinusitis)	Greater yang (*tài yáng*) channel phlegm-damp with wind

$\vee$

Symptom	Disorder
• TEARS: *	
Occurs when facing the wind	'Cold' tears
Feels hot or burning	'Hot' tears
• EYELIDS:	
Bags below the eyes	Spleen weakness leading to accumulation of dampness
Eyelids sticking together	Dampness
• SUBJECTIVE SENSATIONS:	
Darkness or specks when rising from a seat	Blood insufficiency or Gallbladder and Kidney weakness
Poor color perception	Dry Liver†
Floaters	Insufficient qi reaching the eyes
• APPEARANCE:	
Eyeball appears blue	Liver heat affecting the Lungs
Eyeball appears yellow	Jaundice
Eyeball appears red	Heat
Black dots	Intestinal worms

* Cold tears are those which are aggravated by cold air and are usually associated with internal cold, while hot tears are aggravated by hot air and are usually associated with internal heat.

† The term 'dry Liver' is not one of the conditions described in standard TCM texts, but it is one that appears in many Chinese texts. The term refers to a condition of weakness in the Liver, and possibly the Kidneys, where the Kidneys (water) have failed to moisten the Liver such that the Liver (wood) loses its flexibility. This condition is sometimes referred to as dry organs (zào zàng) and sometimes as deficient and weak Liver and Kidneys (gān shèn xū ruò).

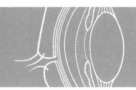

Chapter 4

Causes of Eye Diseases

Eye diseases are nearly always associated with a more extensive pattern affecting the entire body. For this reason, the causes of eye and bodily diseases are the same, for example, overwork and stress. There are a few differences that are discussed here. In addition, there are factors that lead to illness which manifests specifically in the eyes, rather than in other parts of the body.

4.1   External Pathogenic Factors

The external pathogenic factors that affect the eye are mainly heat and dryness; cold and dampness do not seem to affect the eyes so much. A wind-heat attack can present with conjunctivitis. Dryness, particularly when it is associated with dust, results in irritated eyes. Likewise, airborne pollen, which is hot by nature, can irritate the eyes.

Some activities that especially affect the eyes include:

- overuse of the eyes in dim light
- staring for long periods at visual display units (VDUs)
- welder's eyes
- swimming pools
- air conditioning
- fluorescent lights

Overuse of the eyes in dim light

This is less of a problem now than it used to be. In the past, it was especially a problem for lace makers who did very delicate work lit only by a single candle. The light was so poor that they had to concentrate it with small globes filled with water.

Staring for long periods at VDUs

This is a modern scourge. The flickering lights, the out-of-focus images, and the oscillating electrostatic fields have ruined many eyes.

Welder's eyes

Hot metals give off infrared radiation that can be absorbed by the eyes, and individuals who regularly work with hot metals, such as welders, absorb large doses of infrared radiation if they do not wear protective goggles. This can lead to acute conditions, such as a very painful form of conjunctivitis, or chronic conditions, such as cataracts.

Swimming pools

The mixture of chlorine-containing chemicals found in public swimming pools often produces severe irritation of the conjunctiva.[1]

Air conditioning

For those who are prone to dry eyes, the air quality produced by an old air-conditioning system can produce great irritation.

Fluorescent lights

The flickering quality of fluorescent lights, as well as the increased amount of ultraviolet radiation produced by some fluorescent lights, can irritate the eyes.

4.2   The Seven Adverse Emotions

When it comes to chronic eye problems, the usual factors, such as overwork and stress, lay the groundwork for the problem. The factor that causes it to manifest in the eyes is often a subtle emotional disturbance.

Joy

Of course, true joy is not an adverse emotion. What is meant here is 'excess' joy, which we might call overexcitement or overstimulation. Excess joy injures first the blood circulation and then the Heart yang. As a result, the eye can be deprived of nourishment. In the short term, it gives rise to difficulty in focusing and blurred vision; in the long term, the vision becomes dim.

Rage

The saying that the "Liver yang rises up and disturbs the functioning of the eyes" reflects some of the effects of rage on the eyes. The long-term effects of rage are to injure the Liver, which then fails to nourish the eyes. In English there is even an expression, "blinded by rage."

In Chinese medicine it is said that when the Liver does not nourish the eyes, light is not 'harvested' properly, leading to black dots and 'flowers' in the visual field. Presumably, the term 'flowers' means both floaters and the appearance in the visual field of colored objects. In the clinic, acupuncturists see many eye conditions that have a Liver pathology.

Worry

Worry injures the qi and the circulation of essence *(jīng qì)*, leading to a reduction in the nourishment, blood, and qi reaching the eyes such that the eyesight loses its sharpness. Other symptoms may include conditions related to stagnation such as ulcers, styes, and inflammation of the eyelids.

Grief and depression

These emotions lead to depression of qi, which then leads to stagnation and eventually to red eyes. Over time, stagnant qi may turn to fire, which can lead to cataracts. Grief may also impair the circulation of retained water and fluids, leading to swollen and painful eyes. In extreme cases this may develop into dim vision and even blindness.

Fear and panic

These injure the fluids, nutritive qi *(yíng qì)*, yin, and essence, leading to dim vision or even total lack of light perception. Alternatively, it can lead to oversensitivity to light. Panic is also a significant factor in acute glaucoma.

The effect of hidden emotions

The discussion above is based on Chinese texts, and refers to the effects that strong emotions have on the yin and yang organs. Once the organs have been affected, the eyes may also be affected. Another way in which the eyes may be affected is by emotions that are not so outwardly strong, but nevertheless exert a powerful influence. In the clinic the practitioner may find that the eyes will be affected when patients have something in their lives that they do not want to 'look at,' that is, the qi received by the eyes is reduced in those who are denying some unpleasant aspect in their lives.

4.3   Some Foods that Directly Affect the Eyes

Garlic

Overconsumption of garlic can lead to red and sore eyes.

Onions

Onions and garlic have a similar effect, but that of onions is less pronounced. Onions can also increase the need for sleep in some people.

Eggs

Overconsumption of eggs increases the tendency of the body to produce pus and encourages acute purulent conjunctivitis. This tendency is more pronounced in children.

Alcohol

The effects of alcohol on focus and its irritating effect on the conjunctiva are well known!

Carrots

Carrots contain β-carotene, which is broken down into retinol (vitamin A), a component of rhodopsin (visual purple).

Animal and bird liver

This can strengthen the eyes.

Blueberries *(Vaccinium myrtillus)*

These improve night vision. Some writers think that blueberries affect the production of visual purple, while others believe that they assist the optic nerve.

4.4   Some Poisons that Can Affect the Eyes

Poisons are a significant factor in some eye illnesses. Foremost is mercury. The other common chemicals discussed here are lead and phosphorous.

Mercury

Chronic mercury poisoning is surprisingly common. The main cause is continuous inhalation of mercury vapor. This can come either from the external environment or, more commonly, from mercury amalgam fillings. In spite of repeated denial by dental authorities, mercury fillings can cause toxic levels of mercury to build up in the bodies of some unfortunate people. This is more common in the elderly (provided they still have teeth!) because the rate of excretion of mercury decreases with age.

Some of the problems that women experience at menopause can be attributed to mercury. The reason why it is such a problem during menopause is that any mercury that cannot be excreted is stored in the bones. At menopause, there is a quite sudden reduction in bone density, and as the calcium leaves the bones, the mercury that has been stored with it is suddenly released (see Appendix 3).

It should be noted that the mercury from faulty amalgam in the teeth can affect the eyes directly by causing congestion in the flow of fluids in the front of the face, thereby reducing nourishment to the eyes.

From the standpoint of TCM there are three main adverse effects associated with mercury:

1. ACCUMULATION OF PHLEGM

Mercury causes a slow and steady buildup of thick phlegm in the system. This may show in many different ways, including cough, nasal catarrh, and poor digestion, often with a gradually swelling abdomen and bubbly, cloudy urine. If the mercury comes mainly from the teeth, then the initial problems are more likely to appear in the head, with aching gums, enlarged lymph nodes in the neck, tight sensation in the cheek bones, and a characteristic symptom of sneezing in sunlight. There may also be a tendency to develop sores round the lips. Eye diseases associated with the flow of fluids, such as dry eyes and even glaucoma, are aggravated in this way.

2. PROGRESSIVE DEGENERATION OF THE NERVES

Mercury poisoning is characterized by trembling limbs, paralysis, and loss of memory—all indicative of degeneration of the nerves. Eye diseases associated with nerve degeneration, such as macular degeneration, are aggravated in this way. It should be noted that many problems found in the elderly, like Parkinson's disease, have symptoms that are similar to those of mercury poisoning.

3. DYSFUNCTION OF THE EXCRETORY FUNCTION OF THE KIDNEYS

This happens because the mercury gradually builds up in the kidneys and interferes with their function. This may lead to such symptoms as aches and pains in the kidneys, tendency to edema, and accumulation of dampness in general as evidenced by excessive salivation. Eye diseases associated with fluid imbalances, such as chronic glaucoma, can be aggravated in this way.

The imbalances described above are the most common ones, but they are not the only ones. The most common patterns are characterized by cold and dampness, but patients with heat disorders and others with yin deficiency that were caused by mercury poisoning are also seen.

SUMMARY

Mercury mainly affects the eyes by the buildup of thick, viscous phlegm in the body, especially in the nose and head. Thus, mercury poisoning can be associated with all the problems relating to fluids, in particular:

- glaucoma, especially when the intraocular pressure is not especially high
- chronic sore eyes, especially when there is continuous discharge
- corneal erosion
- retinal degeneration

Lead

There are many sources of lead in the environment. In the past, lead was used extensively in plumbing, and there are still a lot of old houses that have lead in the plumbing somewhere. This is especially a danger when the water flowing through the pipes is 'soft,' that is, low in calcium salts.

Until recently, lead in petrol fumes has been a significant cause of lead buildup in the body, and astonishingly, there are countries in Europe that still allow lead to be added to petrol. Lead is, in fact, quite a widespread pollutant, but is generally rather easily excreted. The process of excretion is very much retarded if there are other heavy metals in the body. Thus, it is common to have an accumulation of lead in the system as a result of mercury poisoning. Without the mercury, the body could have eliminated the lead, but with the extra load, especially one that affects the Kidneys and the Large Intestine, the lead accumulates.

In traditional Chinese medicine the main effect of lead can be summed up by saying that it depletes Kidney yang and leads to atrophy disorders *(wei syndrome)*. From the point of view of Western medicine, lead poisoning primarily affects the brain. Typical symptoms are initially progressive weakening of the body, tiredness, pallor, and loss of libido. Later symptoms are weak legs, progressive nervous system degeneration, with paralysis and numbness, loss of memory, and all the grim brain diseases of old age. Again, old people are more likely to suffer because of the progressive difficulty in excreting lead. As with mercury poisoning, the common patterns involve cold and deficiency, but I have seen patients with hot patterns as well.

The effect of lead on the eyes is mainly on the nervous system and retina, causing such symptoms as:

- inflammation of the optic nerve
- optic nerve atrophy
- macular degeneration
- glaucoma

Phosphorous

The main source of excess phosphorous is from agricultural chemicals, particularly pesticides (organophosphates), which are present in food. The main effects of organophosphates are on the nervous system and sensory organs, injuring them while increasing their sensitivity. At first, the only noticeable effect is a tendency to overstimulation and overexcitement. The next stage includes mild yin deficiency symptoms, followed by more severe symptoms such as paralysis.

The effects on the eyes are mainly those associated with yin deficiency:

- oversensitivity to light, requiring sunglasses even at night
- dry, red eyes
- cataracts
- glaucoma
- retinal damage

Endnote

1. The irritation and odor associated with chlorinated swimming pools can be readily reversed by washing with a dilute vitamin C bath.

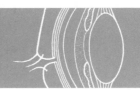

Chapter 5

Acupuncture Points that Affect the Eyes

5.1 Local Points

There are many points that surround the eyes (Fig. 5.1). Most of these can only be needled perpendicularly to a depth of 0.2 to 0.3 units because of the underlying bone. But there are some points, such as BL-1 *(jing ming)*, that can be needled either superficially or deeply. As a general rule, superficial needling affects the front of the eye and is suitable for conditions like conjunctivitis, while deep needling affects the back of the eye and is suitable for conditions such as retinal degeneration.

The reason for needling deeply at points such as BL-1 *(jing ming)*, ST-1 *(cheng qi)*, or M-HN-8 *(qiu hou)* is to obtain a qi sensation at the back of the eye. The deep needling technique is illustrated in Fig. 5.2. Although many practitioners instinctively recoil at the idea of needling so deeply, it is not dangerous to do if it is done carefully. The sclera is one of the toughest parts of the body, and it is nearly impossible to do more harm than scratching it with an acupuncture needle. The main adverse effect of needling is to cause a black eye, but deep needling is no more likely to do so than shallow needling.

Deep needling at these points is necessary during the first few treatments to get the qi sensation to radiate to the back of the eye. As the qi improves, shallower needling is often enough to produce a sensation that will reach there.

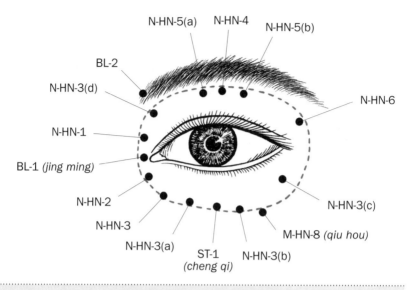

Fig. 5.1 Points surrounding the eye

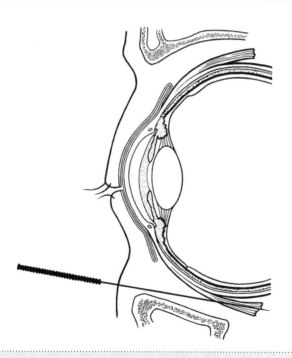

Fig. 5.2 Method for needling ST-1 *(cheng qi)* and M-HN-8 *(qiu hou)*

BL-1 *(jing ming)*

METHOD: This point may be needled superficially or deeply using a perpendicular insertion. The superficial depth is 0.2 to 0.3 units while the deep depth is 1 to 1.5 units. In order to needle deeply, the patient should be asked to look away from the needle so that the pupil is as far as possible from the needle. The eye is then gently pushed further away by the practitioner before needling is begun. After withdrawing the needle, the point should be pressed firmly with a cotton ball to prevent a hematoma.

INDICATIONS: All eye problems.

BL-2 *(zan zhu)*

METHOD: Needle toward BL-1 *(jing ming)*, 0.5 to 1 unit. The sensation should be felt in the eye.

INDICATIONS: All eye problems.

GB-14 *(yang bai)*

METHOD: Oblique insertion, 1 to 1.5 units. Usually needled toward M-HN-6 *(yu yao)*, but may be needled toward either side.

INDICATIONS: Sore eyes, twitching of the eyelid, itching eyelid.

GB-15 *(tou lin qi)*[1]

METHOD: Oblique insertion, 0.5 to 1 unit.

INDICATIONS: Headache, blurred vision, pain in the outer canthus.

ST-1 *(cheng qi)*

METHOD: Needle to 1 to 2 units, first slightly downward, then slightly upward. Before needling, press the eyeball gently upward. The needle is gently eased around the sphere of the eye. If any resistance is felt, the needle should be withdrawn slightly and redirected before continuing. After withdrawing, press the point firmly with a cotton ball to prevent a hematoma.

INDICATIONS: All eye problems.

ST-2 *(si bai)*

METHOD: Straight insertion, 0.2 to 0.3 units, or oblique insertion, 1 unit.

INDICATIONS: Red eyes, corneal opacity.

TB-23 *(si zhu kong)*

METHOD: Needle transversely, 0.5 to 1 unit.

INDICATIONS: red eyes, entropion (in-grown eyelashes).

M-HN-5 *(tou guang ming)*

LOCATION: 0.3 unit directly above M-HN-6 *(yu yao)*.

METHOD: Lateral needling, 0.5 unit.

INDICATIONS: Inability to focus, pain in the eye, cataract.

M-HN-6 *(yu yao)*

LOCATION: In the hollow in the middle of the eyebrow, directly above the pupil of the eye.

METHOD: Needle transversely, 0.5 to 1 unit.

INDICATIONS: Myopia, conjunctivitis, corneal ulcer, corneal opacity, stye, entropion.

M-HN-8 *(qiu hou)*

LOCATION: At the inferior border of the orbit, approximately one-fourth the distance from the lateral to the medial side of the orbit.

METHOD: Needle 1 to 2 units, first slightly downward, then slightly upward (see directions for ST-1 *[cheng qi]*). Note that this point has almost the same actions as ST-1 *(cheng qi)*, but is slightly easier to needle because of the extra space between the bone of the orbit and the sphere of the eyeball.

INDICATIONS: Myopia, inflammation or atrophy of the optic nerve, glaucoma, retinitis pigmentosa, convergent crossed eyes, cataract, recovery after eye surgery, after-effects of a stroke.

N-HN-1 *(shang jing ming)*[2]

LOCATION: 0.2 unit above BL-1 *(jing ming)*.

METHOD: Straight insertion, 1 to 1.5 units.

INDICATIONS: All eye problems, especially optic nerve atrophy.

N-HN-2 *(xia jing ming)*[3]

LOCATION: 0.2 unit below BL-1 *(jing ming)*.

METHOD: Straight insertion, 1 to 1.5 units.

INDICATIONS: Same as for N-HN-1 *(shang jing ming)*.

N-HN-3 *(jian ming)*[4]

LOCATION: 0.2 unit below and slightly lateral to N-NH-2 *(xia jing ming)*.

METHOD: Straight insertion, 1 to 1.5 units.

INDICATIONS: Many eye problems, including retinitis,[5] cataract, and atrophy of the optic nerve.

N-HN-3(a) *(jian ming #1)*

LOCATION: Between N-HN-3 *(jian ming)* and ST-1 *(cheng qi)*.

METHOD: Needle along the margin of the orbit, slightly toward the inner canthus, 1 to 1.5 units.

INDICATIONS: Corneal ulcer, corneal atrophy, cataract.

N-HN-3(b) *(jian ming #2)*

LOCATION: Between ST-1 *(cheng qi)* and M-HN-8 *(qiu hou)*, inside and inferior to the margin of the orbit.

METHOD: Insert along the margin of the orbit, slightly toward the inner canthus, 1 to 1.5 units.

INDICATIONS: Atrophy of the optic nerve, white blobs on the cornea or sclera, corneal opacity.

N-HN-3(c) *(jian ming #3)*

LOCATION: 0.3 unit lateral and superior to M-HN-8 *(qiu hou)*.

METHOD: Needle along the margin of the orbit, slightly toward the inner canthus, 1 to 1.5 units.

INDICATIONS: Same as for N-HN-3(b) *(jian ming #2)*.

N-HN-3(d) *(jian ming #4)*

LOCATION: 0.3 unit above N-HN-1 *(shang jing ming)*.

METHOD: Needle along the margin of the orbit, slightly toward the inner canthus, 1 to 1.5 units.

INDICATIONS: Glaucoma, difficulty in focusing, cataract.

N-HN-4 *(shang ming)*

LOCATION: Directly below the midpoint of the end of eyebrows, just under the superior border of the orbit.

METHOD: Straight insertion along the superior border of the orbit, 1 to 1.5 units.

INDICATIONS: Same as for N-HN-1 *(shang jing ming)*.

N-HN-5(a) *(zeng ming #1)*

LOCATION: 0.2 unit medial to N-HN-4 *(shang ming)*.

METHOD: Insert along the margin of the orbit, slightly toward the inner canthus, 1 to 1.5 units.

INDICATIONS: Corneal opacity, difficulty in focusing.

N-HN-5(b) *(zeng ming #2)*

LOCATION: 0.2 unit lateral to N-HN-4 *(shang ming)*.

METHOD: Same as for N-HN-5(a) *(zeng ming #1)*.

INDICATIONS: Same as for N-HN-5(a) *(zeng ming #1)*.

N-HN-6 *(wai ming)*

LOCATION: 0.3 unit above the outer canthus of the eye.

METHOD: Straight insertion along the superior border of the orbit, 1 to 1.5 units.

INDICATIONS: All eye problems, especially optic nerve atrophy.

GB-1 *(tong zi liao)*

METHOD: Needle laterally, 0.2 to 0.3 unit.

INDICATIONS: Pain in the eye, poor vision, red eye, watering eye.

5.2   Near Points

M-HN-9 *(tai yang)*

METHOD: Either straight insertion, 0.5 to 1 unit; toward the eye, 0.5 to 1 unit; or bleeding with the triangular needle.

INDICATIONS: All eye diseases, especially red and swollen eyes, or stye.

M-HN-10 *(er jian)*

LOCATION: Apex of the ear.

METHOD: Bleed or use 5 moxibustion cones.

INDICATIONS: Painful eyes, corneal opacity.

M-HN-13 *(yi ming)*[6]

LOCATION: 1 unit posterior to TB-17 *(yi feng)*.

METHOD: Straight insertion, 1 to 1.5 units.

INDICATIONS: Far sightedness, near sightedness, cataract, corneal opacity, dim vision, acute glaucoma, optic nerve atrophy, optic neuritis, papilledema.

GV-23 *(shang xing)*

METHOD: Oblique insertion, 0.5 to 1 unit.

INDICATIONS: Eye pain, sore eyes, myopia.

ST-8 *(tou wei)*

METHOD: Upward or downward insertion, 0.5 to 1 unit.

INDICATIONS: Blurred vision, weak or unclear vision, pain in the eyes, excessive tears, spasm of the eyelid.

GB-20 *(feng chi)*

METHOD: Straight insertion, 1 to 1.5 units. When needling this point, it is beneficial to obtain a sensation of warmth in the eye. In the days of the Chinese Cultural Revolution, this point was frequently needled deeply, up to 3 units. This may be done safely if the needle is directed toward the opposite eye. In my experience, it is rarely necessary to needle this deeply in order to get the qi sensation in the eye.

INDICATIONS: All eye diseases.

*xia feng chi**

LOCATION: 0.5 unit below GB-20.

METHOD: Straight insertion, 2 units.

INDICATIONS: Retinal problems, acute glaucoma.

* No alphanumeric code exists for this point.

BL-6 *(cheng guang)*

METHOD: Oblique insertion, 0.3 to 0.5 unit.

INDICATIONS: All eye diseases, especially the presence of a film over the eye.

TB-17 *(yi feng)*[7]

METHOD: Straight insertion, 2 to 2.5 units, toward the nearest eye. Note that when the point is used to treat hearing problems and is needled toward the tongue, the maximum depth is only 1 to 1.5 units. When treating hearing problems, it is beneficial to get a very strong sensation in the ear when needling this point. By contrast, when the point is used to treat eye problems, a more gentle sensation is sufficient. It is helpful if the sensation radiates to the eye.

INDICATIONS: All eye problems, especially corneal opacity.

TB-20 *(jiao sun)*

METHOD: Oblique insertion, 0.3 to 0.5 unit.

INDICATIONS: Redness, pain, swelling of the eyes.

5.3 Distal Points

BL-18 *(gan shu)*[8]

METHOD: Straight insertion, 1 to 1.5 units.

INDICATIONS: Tonifies the Liver and thus is beneficial in all eye diseases.

BL-20 *(pi shu)*

METHOD: Straight insertion, 1 to 1.5 units.

INDICATIONS: Tonifies the Spleen and thus is beneficial in all eye diseases with underlying Spleen weakness. Typically, this includes many chronic conditions with fluid circulation or phlegm imbalance, such as glaucoma or corneal erosion.

BL-23 *(shen shu)*

METHOD: Straight insertion, 1 to 1.5 units.

INDICATIONS: Tonifies the Kidneys and thus is beneficial in all eye diseases with Kidney weakness. Typically, this includes optic nerve and fluid circulation problems.

LR-2 *(xing jian)*

METHOD: Straight insertion, 0.5 to 1 unit.

INDICATIONS: Clears heat from the Liver and thus is beneficial for red and painful eye disorders, as well as many other eye conditions.

LR-3 *(tai chong)*

METHOD: Needle toward KI-1 *(yong quan)*, 1 to 1.5 units. The dispersing method is used to reduce rising Liver yang, while the tonifying method is used for all conditions of Liver weakness. To tonify both the Liver and Kidneys, this point may be needled even more deeply so that the sensation is felt in the sole of the foot. To produce a tonifying effect, the needling should be done gently.

INDICATIONS: Tonifies the Liver and thus benefits the free flow of qi, especially for painful eyes and chronic eye diseases.

GB-37 *(guang ming)*

METHOD: Straight insertion, 1 to 1.5 units.

INDICATIONS: Night blindness, atrophy of the optic nerve, cataract, pain and itching in the eyes.

TB-2 *(ye men)*

METHOD: Straight insertion, 0.2 to 0.3 unit.

INDICATIONS: Red or sore eyes, such as after a long flight or when sleep deprived.

TB-3 *(zhong zhu)*

METHOD: Straight insertion, 1 to 1.5 units.

INDICATIONS: Red eyes, blurred vision.

SI-6 *(yang lao)*

METHOD: Needle toward PC-6 *(nei guan)*; many books give the heroic depth of 1 to 1.5 units, but such deep needling is not always necessary. Moxibustion can also be done here.

INDICATIONS: Blurred vision, glaucoma (moxibustion).

LI-4 *(he gu)*

METHOD: Straight insertion, 1 to 1.5 units.

INDICATIONS: Beneficial for all eye diseases,[9] especially those affecting the anterior part of the eye, such as conjunctivitis.

ST-36 *(zu san li)*

METHOD: Straight insertion, 1 to 2 units.

INDICATIONS: All deficiency conditions.

ST-44 *(nei ting)*

METHOD: Needle toward the ankle, 0.3 to 0.8 unit.

INDICATIONS: Eye pain, all problems of the anterior part of the eye.

M-UE-15 *(da gu kong)*[10]

LOCATION: On the dorsal surface, at the center of the phalangeal joint of the thumb (Fig. 5.3).

METHOD: Moxibustion stick for 5 to 10 minutes or 3 to 7 moxibustion cones.

INDICATIONS: All eye diseases, especially chronic pain in the eye, glaucoma, cataracts, and nebula;[11] also for vomiting, diarrhea, arthritic pain in the thumb.

M-UE-17 *(xiao gu kong)*[12]

LOCATION: On the top of the proximal end of the second phalangeal bone of the little finger (Fig. 5.4).

METHOD: Moxibustion stick for 5 to 10 minutes or 3 to 7 moxibustion cones.

INDICATIONS: All eye diseases; also for arthritic pain of the little finger.

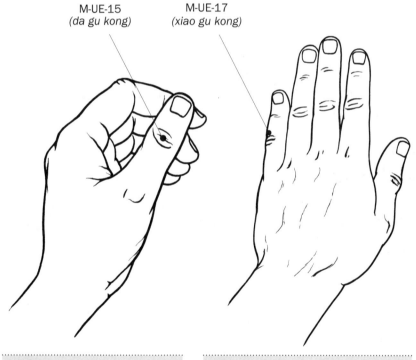

M-UE-15
(da gu kong)

M-UE-17
(xiao gu kong)

Fig. 5.3
Location of M-UE-15 *(da gu kong)*

Fig. 5.4
Location of M-UE-17 *(xiao gu kong)*

Endnotes

1. *Tóu* means 'head.'

2. *Shàng* means 'upper'.

3. *Xià* means 'lower'.

4. *Jiàn* means 'healthy' or 'strengthen'. The point is also known as *jiàn yáng*.

5. Retinitis indicates an inflammation of the retina; the term was used in the older ophthalmological literature to indicate impairment of sight, edema, and exudation or hemorrhages affecting the retina.

6. *Yì míng* means 'shielding brightness' or 'shade brightness.' The character *yì* is a technical term used in TCM ophthalmology to indicate dimness of vision.

7. *Yì fēng* means 'shielding wind' or 'shade wind.'

8. BL-18 *(gan shu)*, BL-20 *(pi shu)*, and BL-23 *(shen shu)* are back associated *(shu)* points.

9. Starting from LI-4 *(he gu)*, the Large Intestine channel joins the Stomach channel on the face and then enters the eyes.

10. *Dà gǔ kōng* means 'big bone hollow'. The point is also called *yan dian san*.

11. Nebula is a superficial corneal opacity.

12. *Xiǎo gǔ kōng* means 'little bone hollow'.

Chapter 6

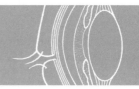

Treatment Principles and Techniques

6.1 Treatment Principles

By the time patients come to acupuncture for the treatment of eye conditions, they are usually quite ill, that is to say, they have an imbalance on more than one level. Typically, the following factors come together to cause an eye disease:

1. Marked reduction of qi in the eyes as a result of a local qi deficiency, and often a general qi deficiency as well.
2. Significant organ imbalance or weakness, for example, Kidney yang deficiency.
3. Attitude problems and life problems, for example, not wanting to look at relationships with nearest and dearest.

These three factors, therefore, provide the basis for treatment.

Bringing qi to the eyes

With acupuncture, this is relatively straightforward. In fact, acupuncture is superior to almost every other therapy in this respect. We have a choice of three classes of points: local, near, and distal. With good needle technique, qi can be directed from the distal and near points to the eyes.

Then there are the local points themselves. Not only do we have the superficial points that surround the orbit, but also the points such as M-HN-8 *(qiu hou)* that can bring qi right to the back of the eyeball, the retina, and the optic nerve. No other therapy comes near acupuncture in this regard!

Treating organ imbalances

By the time patients come to us with a degenerative eye disease, the organs have become significantly depleted. This can be addressed with acupuncture and many other therapies. Because of the nature of the illnesses, back-associated *(shu)* points are frequently used.

Changing the patient's attitude

This part is the most difficult, regardless of the treatment modality. For example, individuals who have reached their late fifties, who feel that they have no future in life, and who have the huge burden of looking after ailing relations may well be without hope. They may well not want to look at their lives and their futures. They may well not wish to face their problems when they wake up in the morning.

Here acupuncture has a slight advantage over herbs because there seems to be something very beneficial to the spirit about this form of treatment. This, after all, is the basis for the five-phase approach to acupuncture, which has so many champions. The results are not quick, of course, but there are results.

Pulling it all together

To summarize, treatment should focus on:

1. *Bringing qi to the eyes.* This is often not as easy as it sounds. For example, while it is true that a few treatments may be sufficient to treat nearsightedness (myopia), in the case of optic nerve atrophy, a large number of treatments—perhaps 50 to 100 daily treatments—may be required.
2. *Treating the overall body condition.* If the organs and the qi of the entire body are weak, then there is not much point in attempting to bring qi to the eyes. If there is no qi in the body, then there is no qi to bring to the eyes. However, when the organs are strong, for example, the eye disorder is a result not of weakness but, say, of Liver yang rising, then this step may be achieved quite quickly.

3. *Changing the patient's attitude.* If a person is still depressed, miserable, angry, or hopeless, then one of the root causes of the illness is still present. Thus, however much qi is brought to the eyes and however strong the organs, the problem is likely to recur the moment the treatment stops.

In some sense, the treatments described in this book may appear simplistic. The same points are listed again and again for widely differing conditions. It would seem that acupuncture is very easy. And in one sense, this is true. Acupuncture *is* very easy, but as any acupuncturist will relate, it is not quite as easy as all that!

The easy part of treatment is the one described in this book, which is to bring qi to the eyes. The difficult part is actually curing the patient, leading her from a condition where the eyes are deteriorating to one where the eyes are improving. This is the true art of acupuncture. A cure of this kind involves helping the patient find a new way to live her life without her illness. This may be difficult, for many patients have become accustomed to being ill and even subconsciously need their illness in some way.

6.2   Treatment Techniques

Besides conventional acupuncture and moxibustion, there are a number of other techniques that can be of benefit, including

- electric plum blossom technique
- traditional Chinese massage
- the Bates' method
- walnut shell spectacles
- microcurrent electrical circulation

Electric plum blossom technique

The phrase sounds a bit like the name of a punk rock group, but the new technique is in fact a happy combination of an old technique and new technology. The plum blossom needle consists of seven sewing-gauge needles tightly bound together. It is called 'plum blossom' because of its resemblance to the stamens of the plum blossom.

The plum blossom needle is a folk instrument since it is easily made, and it is used in many homes in China in much the same way that people in the West use aspirin or paracetamol for aches, pains, head colds, and the flu. Treatment is given by a steady tapping on the skin until it is slightly red, or even slightly bleeding. Sometimes whole areas are tapped, for example, along the channel for rheumatic pain in the legs. At other times individual points are tapped, for example, GB-20 *(feng chi)* and LI-4 *(he gu)* for head colds. It is a very simple and effective treatment technique. However, it has not caught on in the West because it causes pain, and Western patients dislike pain.

Fortunately, with the aid of modern technology, the plum blossom needle can be used without causing pain. This is achieved by using the electrical stimulation provided by an old-fashioned acupuncture point stimulator, or TENS[1] machine. Electricity is much more controllable than mechanical hammering, and the combination of the plum blossom needle and the TENS machine should not cause any pain. It is especially suited to the points around the eyes where the skin is delicate and sensitive. The technique is used to stimulate the acupuncture points as follows:

1. Lay the plum blossom needle on the point to be stimulated and connect the positive electrode to it. The patient holds the (negative) electrode in the other hand.
2. Gradually increase the electrical stimulation. At first, the patient will feel nothing. Then the patient will feel a slight tingle and, finally, a buzzing, warm, distended feeling. It should be a pleasant sensation, somewhat akin to a pleasant qi sensation.
3. Maintain this sensation for 10 to 20 seconds.
4. Remove the plum blossom needle and turn down the electricity, to prepare for the next point.

Traditional Chinese massage

This method is gentle and is widely taught in Chinese schools to prevent children from becoming shortsighted from too much reading and other visual activity. For mild eye problems, such as tired eyes or mildly itching eyes, these simple massage techniques can be of great benefit. In severe cases, massage is a useful supplement to other, stronger therapies. The following massages should be done three times a day.

MASSAGING ABOVE THE EYES

Make a fist, with the thumb bent at its middle joint. Use this joint to massage above the eyes, 30 times (Fig. 6.1 and 6.2).

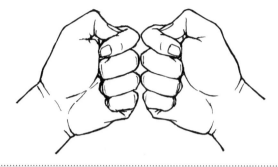

Fig. 6.1 How to hold the thumbs

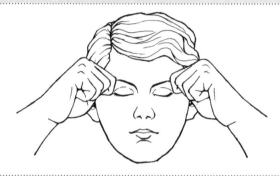

Fig. 6.2 Massaging the eyebrows

PINCHING AND PRESSING BL-1 *(jing ming)*

The pinching should be done with a vibrating movement, about 50 times (Fig. 6.3).

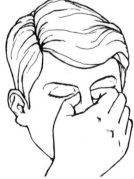

Fig. 6.3 Pinching and pressing BL-1 *(jing ming)*

MASSAGING M-HN-9 (tai yang)

Massage with the tips of the fingers about 50 times (Fig. 6.4).

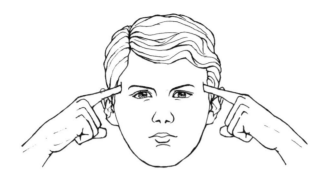

Fig. 6.4   Massaging M-HN-9 (tai yang)

MASSAGING GB-20 (feng chi)

Both thumbs should be pressed in firmly and rotated about 50 times. This point is often sore but should be massaged until the soreness goes away (Fig. 6.5).

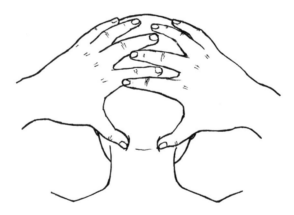

Fig. 6.5   Massaging GB-20 (feng chi)

MASSAGING LI-4 (he gu)

The thumb of the opposite hand is pressed in and vibrated or rotated about 50 times. Repeat on the other hand (Fig. 6.6).

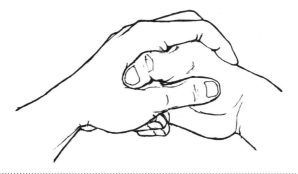

Fig. 6.6   Massaging LI-4 *(he gu)*

The Bates' method

This is not the place to give a full description of the Bates' method. It has been done well in many other publications. However, this is a wonderful method that has saved thousands of people's eyesight. Put very simply, the goal of this method is to train the eyes to look properly. The basis of the method is that all eye problems derive from faulty habits of using the eyes, so that by developing good habits, the eyes will be self-nourishing and self-invigorating.

Bates himself trained a number of people in his technique. Now, there are many teachers of the Bates' method.

Walnut shell spectacles

These are spectacles where each lens has been replaced by a half walnut shell (Fig. 6.7). The method is to soak the shells in a strong decoction of chrysanthemum flowers overnight before placing them in the frames. Then place a short length of moxibustion stick one inch (2.5cm) or so in front of the shells, which warms them up. The combination of the warmth from the shells and the vapor from the chrysanthemum extract is very soothing to the eyes.

This technique is effective for bringing qi to the eyes and is of special use in treating tired eyes and chronic red eyes. It can also be used as a supplemental treatment technique in all eye conditions. At the time of writing, there are very few suppliers of these spectacles, and the practitioner would be advised to make them out of stout low-conductivity wire.

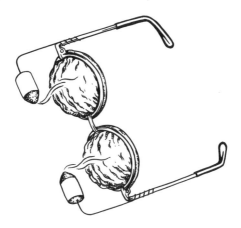

Fig. 6.7 Walnut shell spectacles

Microcurrent electrical stimulation

This is a promising new development of an old technique, electrical stimulation of acupuncture points. It could be said to be an improved version of the electrical plum blossom method. The difference between the two methods is that the electrical plum blossom method is normally used with a rather old-fashioned type of stimulator that operates at a constant voltage and a relatively low frequency. The amount of current therefore varies with the skin resistance. By contrast, the microcurrent electrical stimulator is delivered by a constant-current device at a much higher frequency (around 15 kHz).

The microcurrent electrical stimulator has an advantage over the older devices in that the current can be controlled easily, and it is the current that does the stimulation. There is an added advantage in using a relatively high-frequency stimulator: electrical currents at high frequencies have the unexpected property that they run along surfaces of discontinuity in conductivity (Fig. 6.8). By contrast, the current generated by low-frequency stimulators passes along the line of least resistance, which is approximately a straight line between the two electrodes.

In the clinic, this means that the electricity can penetrate very deeply at low currents. In particular, it means that a gentle stimulation at the skin adjacent to the eye will penetrate all the way around the eyeball to the retina at the back. This is an enormously useful tool, for it means that stimulation can be given to the eye non-invasively. To do the same with an acupuncture needle is possible, but it involves deep insertion (1.2–2 inches/30–50mm) in points like ST-1 *(cheng qi)* or M-HN-8 *(qiu hou).* It requires a skilled practitioner to do this without injuring nearby tissue. Placing the electrode on the skin and giving an electrical stimulation needs no skill and can be done by the patient himself, allowing treatments several times a day.

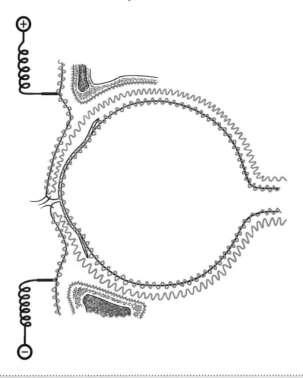

Fig. 6.8 Path taken by high-frequency current

Some research has been done on this phenomenon, and it has been found that there are two types of stimulation, very similar to the needle techniques of tonifying and dispersing.[2] If strong stimulation—stimulation that is relatively painful—is given, it has the effect of reducing the activity of cells. If weak stimulation—stimulation that is well below the pain threshold—is given, it has the effect of invigorating underactive cells. To obtain a weak stimulation, the current is increased to the point that the patient just feels the stimulation. The current is then reduced so that the patient no longer feels anything.

The uses of this technique have been pioneered by Dr. Damon Miller in the treatment of macular degeneration. At the time of writing this book, information concerning these uses is provided on his website at *www.acupunctureworks. com.*

Endnotes

1. TENS is an acronym for transcutaneous electrical nerve stimulator.

2. Personal communication with Dr. Damon Miller.

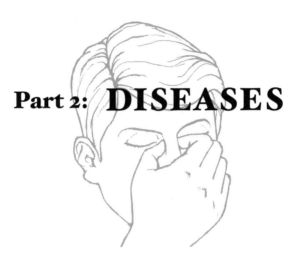

Part 2: DISEASES

Chapter 7

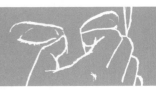

Retinal Problems Leading to Loss of Vision

This chapter deals with retinal problems that have loss of vision as their major presentation (Fig. 7.1). Section 7.1 covers four eye diseases that were traditionally grouped together, largely because progressive loss of vision is their primary clinical symptom. The grouping together of these disorders is not based, however, on a common etiology as understood by Western medicine. This section does not include open-angle glaucoma, which also leads to progressive loss of vision, since this condition is discussed in Chapter 8. Section 7.2 covers two eye diseases, one of which may result in a rather sudden loss of vision, while the other does not. Localized edema is found in both conditions.

7.1 Optic Atrophy, Macular Degeneration, Retinitis Pigmentosa, and Night Blindness

Etiology and symptoms

Optic atrophy

Optic atrophy is the name given to progressive loss of function, in other words atrophy, of the optic nerve (Fig. 7.2). From the patient's point of view, it is experienced as progressive blindness, which can involve either the peripheral or central vision. Optic atrophy can result in total blindness with a pupil that is unreactive to light. There are a number of causes of this condition, which include problems in the blood supply to the eye (for example, arterial occlusion), retrobulbar neuritis, retinitis pigmentosa, compression by an adjacent tumor, or glaucoma. Optic atrophy is therefore a catch-all phrase.

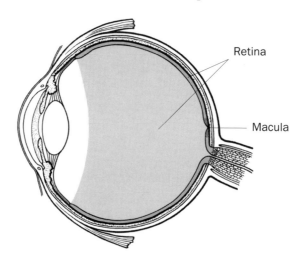

Fig. 7.1 The retina and macula

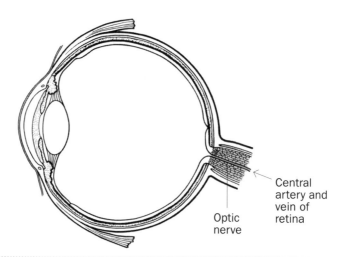

Fig. 7.2 The optic nerve and central artery

Macular degeneration

The macula is the central part of the retina, the part that receives the most finely detailed information, since, notwithstanding its small size, it contains a large fraction of the daylight-sensitive and color-sensitive photoreceptor cells. Macular degeneration is the name given to degradation of the macula that results in deterioration in the central field of vision.[1] The symptoms of macular degeneration include:

- the need for increasingly bright illumination for close work
- a blind spot in the center of the field of vision
- colors that seem washed out
- a gradual increase in the haziness of the overall vision

In some ways, macular degeneration is similar to open-angle glaucoma in that blind patches develop slowly in both conditions. In glaucoma, the blind patches develop from the exterior of the field of vision while in macular degeneration the blindness develops at the center. Since, in macular degeneration, it is the central field of vision that first becomes impaired, the patient quickly becomes aware of the condition. By contrast, in glaucoma, the patient may not be aware of the changes in the peripheral field of vision until the condition is well advanced.

Macular degeneration leads to progressive blindness, but there is an end to the disease. Untreated, macular degeneration continues until most of the macula has ceased to function, but then it stops. This means that even in the late stages of the disease, patients are partially sighted, not completely blind. Their peripheral vision remains so that, although they cannot read, they can nevertheless get around the home and do many daily chores using their peripheral vision.

Retinitis pigmentosa

The name 'retinitis' is a misnomer, for it implies some degree of inflammation of the retina, which is not present in this condition. Retinitis pigmentosa is usually experienced by the patient as a gradual loss of peripheral vision, although there are some cases of the central vision degenerating first, leading eventually to tunnel vision. On examination, it is found that the retina has areas of deep pigmentation. Why this happens is not fully understood, but it is thought to be due to abnormal growth of epithelial cells. This is accompanied by progressive reduction in the number of active retinal cells, which is considered irreversible.

NIGHT BLINDNESS

Night blindness (nyctalopia), or an inability to see anything at all in the dark, is a symptom to be taken very seriously for it is often the precursor to optic atrophy and full blindness. Night blindness is sometimes the result of an inadequate intake or use of vitamin A. If this is the case, other symptoms associated with vitamin A deficiency, such as dryness of the cornea and conjunctiva, 'thickening' of the lungs, digestive tract, and/or urinary tract, and increased susceptibility to infections, can often also be present.

TCM approach

The three diseases—optic atrophy, macular degeneration, and retinitis pigmentosa—are diagnosed differently by Western medical professionals. However, to TCM practitioners, they are all treated identically since they are all disorders of the nervous system, either of the optic nerve itself or of the retina, which is an extension of the nervous system. From the point of view of TCM, what is critical is not so much which part of the nervous system is degrading, but rather that the system itself is degrading and the vision is being impaired as a result. More important than the details of how the illness manifests is the underlying imbalance that has caused the problem in the first place.

These illnesses are similar—in their patterns and in their level of difficulty in treatment—to those illnesses that are classified as atrophy disorders *(wei syndrome)* by TCM practitioners. A quick look at the underlying common condition—a degeneration of the nervous system—will explain why. Nerves are very slow to regenerate at the best of times. (Until recently, it was thought that they did not regenerate at all.) In addition, these illnesses tend to affect older people so there is little energy left in the body to initiate the healing process; often the elderly's very approach to life is part of the problem, and can therefore only be changed with difficulty. This all adds up to diseases that are difficult to cure. However, on the bright side, regular treatment can do wonders in reducing or even halting the progress of the diseases.

CAUSES

Physical causes

The fundamental cause of these problems is exhaustion of the body. This may come from old age, overwork, heart weakness, or, in some cases, deficiency from a long-term diet of poor-quality food ('junk food'). These factors may be combined with a general lack of health as a result of not exercising. This accounts for the first three patterns listed below, namely Liver and Kidney weakness, Spleen and Kidney yang deficiency, and Heart *ying* (nourishment) deficiency.

In all the cases I have seen, there has been some measure of exhaustion but not enough to cause blindness. From this I have deduced that there is another factor at work, which may be heavy metal poisoning, such as mercury poisoning from amalgam fillings in the teeth. Commonly, this is combined with emotional states that reduce the flow of qi to the eyes.

Emotional causes

We have mentioned previously that those who suffer from the various forms of optic atrophy may not want to *see* something that is of great importance in their lives. They are relying on the well-known human behavior—if you ignore something, perhaps it will go away. This approach sometimes works, but here it has not worked, and they have been doing it for a long time. Common problems that obstinately refuse to go away are described in the following table:

Fear of death	This is quite a natural fear, and there must be only a few of us who are not afraid. What tends to cause optical problems is when there is denial of the fear or denial of even the possibility of death. This may come, for example, from a belief in rationalism and a complete rejection of anything spiritual.
Difficult life circumstances	There are many difficult circumstances in life, some of which cannot be changed. An example that may give rise to eye problems can be seen in an individual who is looking after a partner whose health and mind is slowly degenerating 'before the [partner's] eyes.' The individual may prefer to live in the past and remember the wonderful person the partner used to be. The emotional attitude may be aggravated by physical exhaustion from the hard work of caring for the partner.
Loneliness	A person who has lost a partner or who has lived a full life in the past may spend most of the time looking back over life and dreaming of how life was better in the past, rather than living in the present.

The main patterns relating to optic atrophy are given in the table below. Of these, the first four are mentioned in many Chinese texts, but the last one is not. It is based on my own experience with Western patients.

Patterns	Signs and Symptoms
Liver and Kidney weakness	Old and tired of life No reserves of strength Weak back May also have incontinence, prostate problems, or uterine prolapse Weak memory
Heart nourishment deficiency	Palpitations Insomnia Easily worried Face white or pale purple May have hardened arteries
Spleen and Kidney yang deficiency	Tired Limbs feel heavy Weak digestion Weak back
Qi and blood stagnation	Frustration Strong feelings, but may be hidden under a cheerful face Purple tongue
Accumulation of phlegm	Face is shiny or looks powdered Tight, compressed feeling in the eyes and face Pulse is slippery or deep

Having mentioned these different patterns, it must be said that all of them have much in common, and the differences are a matter of emphasis. So, for example, patients with a Heart nourishment deficiency pattern are quite likely to have significant problems in the circulation of blood in the eyes, for example, degeneration of the arteries or even blood stagnation. However, even patients with Liver and Kidney weakness, where the main problem is not arterial, are quite likely to have at least *some* disturbance in the blood supply to the eyes and at least *some* hardening of the arteries.

There is another characteristic shared by these patients, and that is the flat, dejected aura that surrounds them. It is not surprising that patients become flat and dejected on learning that they are going blind, but the emotional problem may predate the physical. The flatness is very much part of the disease, the reason being that this sort of disease can only happen when there is a reduction of qi *coming out* of the eyes. The eyes are not only a conduit for light to enter the body; they are also a conduit for Kidney qi, modified by the spirit, to leave the body. Looking is not a passive function; it is active. So if a person is going blind in this manner, it means that insufficient Kidney qi is reaching the eyes. This is true regardless of the Western medical diagnosis—optic atrophy or macular degeneration—and this is one of the reasons why these illnesses are so hard to cure.

Treatment

The text below is divided into treatment of the main points and treatment according to the pattern.

▶ *Main Points*

Local points	BL-1 (jing ming)	Brings qi to the eyes
	M-HN-8 (qiu hou)	Brings qi to the eyes
Near point	GB-20 (feng chi)	Brings qi to the eyes
Distal points	ST-36 (zu san li)	Tonifies the overall qi
	LR-3 (tai chong)	Benefits the eyes

METHOD: When needling local points, such as BL-1 *(jing ming)*, ST-1 *(cheng qi)*, and M-HN-8 *(qiu hou)*, the sensation should reach the back of the eye. Ideally, there should be a warm, comfortable sensation associated with the needling. In the later stages of treatment, when the qi is flowing well, these points need only be needled to a depth of 0.5 unit for the qi sensation to reach to the back of the eye. However, in the early stages of treatment, it may be necessary to needle to a heroic depth of 2 units before any sensation is felt at the back of the eye. See Fig. 5.2 for further information on needling these sensitive points.

When needling near points, such as GB-20 *(feng chi)*, again the ideal is to get the sensation going to the eye. However, these points should be used even if the patient can experience a qi sensation only locally.

▶ *Liver and Kidney Weakness*

TREATMENT PRINCIPLE: Strengthen the Liver and Kidneys.

BL-23 (*shen shu*)	Tonifies and strengthens the Liver and Kidneys
KI-3 (*tai xi*)	Strengthens Kidney yin
GB-37 (*guang ming*)	Nourishes the Liver and brightens the eyes
LR-3 (*tai chong*)	Nourishes the Liver and brightens the eyes

METHOD: These points are tonified.

▶ *Heart Nourishment Deficiency*

TREATMENT PRINCIPLE: Strengthen the Heart.
In addition to the main points, add:

HT-7 (*shen men*)	Source (*yuan*) point of the Heart
BL-15 (*xin shu*)	Back associated (*shu*) point of the Heart

METHOD: These points are tonified.

▶ *Spleen and Kidney Yang Deficiency*

TREATMENT PRINCIPLE: Tonify the Spleen and Kidneys.
In addition to the main points, add:

ST-36 (*zu san li*)	Tonifies the Stomach, Spleen, and Kidneys
SP-6 (*san yin jiao*)	Strengthens the Spleen, Kidneys, and Liver

METHOD: These points are tonified.

▶ *Qi and Blood Stagnation*

TREATMENT PRINCIPLE: Move stagnant blood.
In addition to the main points, add:

LR-2 (*xing jian*)	Disperses Liver blood
SP-6 (*san yin jiao*)	Brightens the eyes and moves the qi and blood

METHOD: These points are treated with the moving or dispersing technique.

▶ *Accumulation of Phlegm*

TREATMENT PRINCIPLE: Resolve the phlegm.
In addition to the main points, add:

ST-40 (*feng long*)	Resolves phlegm
GB-34 (*yang ling quan*)	Resolves phlegm

METHOD: These points are treated with the even technique. For this pattern it may be more appropriate to use moxibustion, especially on local points around the eyes. The use of walnut shell spectacles (see Section 6.2) are also recommended here.

COMMENT

Most of the patients that I have seen have had the Western medical diagnosis of macular degeneration, and they did not have an easily recognizable TCM pattern. Rather, they had a mixture of all five patterns, with weakness predominant. When this occurs, the principle of treatment is first to bring qi to the eyes and then to tonify, with points such as the following:

ST-36 (*zu san li*)	Tonifies the source qi
SP-6 (*san yin jiao*)	Tonifies the Liver and Kidneys
BL-23 (*shen shu*)	Tonifies the Kidneys
BL-18 (*gan shu*)	Tonifies the Liver
BL-20 (*pi shu*)	Tonifies the Liver and Spleen

FREQUENCY OF TREATMENT

There are two aspects to the treatment: bringing qi to the eyes and improving the overall body condition so that there is more qi to bring to the eyes.

- *Bringing qi to the eyes.* This is done by needling the local points and ideally should be done once a day in the early stages. At the very least, it should be done three times a week for any significant result. If this is impossible, a good second best is to do the eye massage techniques described in Section 6.2 three times a day, or perform microcurrent electrical stimulation, also discussed in Section 6.2, once or more a day.
- *Treating the overall body condition.* This part of the treatment involves strengthening any weakness of the organs, a process that inevitably takes time. Treatment once or twice a week is all that is needed. Thus, a practical combination is for the patient to visit the practitioner once a week for treating the overall condition, while performing daily local treatments at home.

RESULTS

The results vary from patient to patient and depend on the severity of the problem, the duration of the condition, the patient's energy, and the possibility of change. If treatment is sufficiently frequent, then, at the very least, degeneration can be halted. If there is retinal degeneration, it can be reversed to some extent, although it is rare to reverse it completely. I have seen some tens of patients with macular degeneration, and the main problem that I found was getting them to come for enough treatments. Those who could come several times a week showed marked improvement.

RESULTS IN A SMALL CLINICAL STUDY

In a report from *Abstracts of Clinical Experience with Acupuncture* (p. 307), acupuncture was used to treat many cases of optic atrophy, macular degeneration, and retinitis pigmentosa. The following points were used:

Local points	BL-1 (*jing ming*)
	ST-1 (*cheng qi*)
Near points	GB-20 (*feng chi*)
	M-HN-13 (*yi ming*)
Distal points	TB-5 (*wai guan*)
	SI-6 (*yang lao*)
	LI-4 (*he gu*)

Needling of the local points was done in such a way that the sensation was felt in the optic nerve. Improvement was noted in 40 to 60 percent of the patients.

Western medical and acupuncture treatments

At present, there are no effective Western medical treatments for these conditions. Acupuncture and microcurrent stimulation (see below) are the treatments of choice, although other treatments such as herbs and homeopathy can also be beneficial.

Other treatments

MICROCURRENT ELECTRICAL STIMULATION

Daily electrical stimulation of the points around the eye with a microcurrent electrical stimulator has been shown to be very beneficial. At the time of writing this book, there is a program under way in California using this method, and good results are being obtained. It appears that everyone who has used the microcurrent electrical stimulator has had beneficial results. There is a disadvantage in that they may need to keep using the stimulator several times a week, for many years, in order to maintain improvement.

The results are consistent with what was said in Chapter 6 in that there are two parts to every treatment. One part is to bring qi to the eyes, which is relatively easy. The other part is to cure the underlying condition, which is relatively difficult. The local stimulation of points brings the qi to the eyes but does little to change the underlying condition.

ADVICE

- It can be helpful to take mineral and vitamin supplements. A broad-spectrum supplement is adequate.
- The patient should be tested for mercury and other heavy metal poisoning (see Appendix 3).

7.2   Optic Neuritis and Papilledema

Both of these illnesses affect the optic nerve (see Fig. 7.2). In addition, both illnesses are characterized by edema, especially in the early stages. In the case of papilledema, the edematous swelling is the cause of the illness.

Etiology and symptoms

OPTIC NEURITIS

Optic neuritis is an inflammation of a part of the optic nerve that can be seen by an ophthalmoscope. The inflammation can be a result of a variety of triggers, including multiple sclerosis,[2] certain chemicals such as lead, syphilis, an inflammation of the arteries,[3] or the aftermath of a bee sting. The condition is often one-sided. Other causes are not known, although it has been noted that in some patients the vision often gets worse after ingesting food, while in others it gets worse after exercising.

Localized bleeding and edema are seen in the early stages of the disease. The symptom can vary from loss of vision in a small portion of the central field to complete blindness. The disease is often rapid and may result in blindness in as little as 24 hours. In the early stages of the disease, successful removal of the cause or even spontaneous remission can result in restoration of the vision.

PAPILLEDEMA

The illness is a result of a swelling of the optic nerve head as a result of increased pressure in the cranium from, for example, encephalitis, severe hypertension, trauma to the head, or emphysema; the condition is almost always bilateral. If the cause of the increase in pressure is not reduced, optic atrophy and a loss of vision will eventually result.

TCM approach

The main patterns relating to optic neuritis are given in the table below. Of these patterns, it is likely that the Stomach heat pattern would be aggravated by food, while the pattern of injured Heart and spirit may well get worse after exercise. What seems to be missing from the Chinese texts is multiple sclerosis, and the probable reason is that this illness is very rare in China.

Pattern	Cause	Signs and Symptoms
Liver yang rising	Restraint of emotions Overwork	Suppressed anger may lead to sudden blindness May have feelings of nausea Facial color may be red or occasionally gray Wiry pulse Purple tongue with thick coating
Heart and spirit injured	Fright, shock, or fear	Emotional trauma may lead to sudden blindness Facial color pale May have blue lips Looks frightened or as though would burst into tears Pulse is unsteady
Stomach heat	Alcohol Spicy foods	Red face Voracious appetite Restless, impatient Tongue body is red and may have thick yellow coating Pulse rapid and slippery

TREATMENT

The discussion below is divided into treatment of the main points and treatment according to the pattern.

▶ Main Points

BL-1 (*jing ming*)	Brings qi to the eyes
M-HN-8 (*qiu hou*)	Brings qi to the eyes

METHOD: Deep needling is required so that the sensation is felt at the back of the eyes. When first needled, the sensation may be similar to that of an electric shock or being stabbed with a knife, either of which may alarm the patient. This sensation is a result of local stagnation being suddenly cleared. After this initial strong sensation, the needle should be very gently manipulated with the tonifying method so that the patient feels a warm sensation at the back of the eye.

▶ Liver Yang Rising

TREATMENT PRINCIPLE: Bring down Liver yang and calm the anger.
In addition to the main points, add:

LR-3 (*tai chong*)	Calms Liver qi
LR-2 (*xing jian*)	Calms Liver fire
LI-4 (*he gu*)	Calms Liver qi

METHOD: These points are treated with a strong dispersing technique.

▶ Heart and Spirit Injured

TREATMENT PRINCIPLE: Strengthen the Heart and calm the spirit.
In addition to the main points, add:

GB-13 (*ben shen*)	Calms the spirit
HT-7 (*shen men*)	Strengthens the Heart and calms the spirit
BL-15 (*xin shu*)	Strengthens the Heart and calms the spirit
KI-3 (*tai xi*)	Tonifies the Kidneys to support the Heart

METHOD: These points are treated using the even or tonifying technique. Lie the patient down when needling KI-3 (*tai xi*) to avoid the risk of fainting.

▶ *Stomach Heat*

TREATMENT PRINCIPLE: Clear Stomach heat.
In addition to the main points, add:

ST-44 (*nei ting*)	Clears Stomach heat
ST-45 (*li dui*)	Clears Stomach heat

METHOD: These points are treated with the dispersing technique.

COMMENT

Although the patterns described are those of excess, the patient may in fact be very tired and weak; the pattern of excess is superimposed on a state of deep exhaustion. If this is the case, then add the following points:

BL-18 (*gan shu*)	Strengthens the Liver
BL-23 (*shen shu*)	Strengthens the Kidneys

METHOD: These points are tonified.

RESULTS

In *Abstracts of Clinical Experience with Acupuncture* (p. 306), acupuncture at local points was used to treat 23 eyes with acute optic neuritis. The results were that four eyes were cured, five were much improved, six showed slight improvement, and eight showed no change.

A note about multiple sclerosis

In order to treat patients with optic neuritis successfully, the practitioner may have to treat the underlying cause: multiple sclerosis. In my experience, multiple sclerosis is an odd disease, often seeming to be a condition of excess when it is really a condition of deficiency, even in the early stages. Patients may be in their 30s or younger and seem full of strength. I have even known cases where the face was red, the pulse was wiry, and the patient exuded an air of repressed anger. Not all cases are so extreme, but it is common to see clear signs of the excess pattern of Liver stagnation.

The obvious treatment in such conditions would be to disperse: the more 'excessive' the patient appears to be, the more dispersal would be indicated. However, it has been my experience, on some tens of patients, that multiple sclerosis patients should always be tonified, whatever the stage of their disease. Even the apparently excessive conditions should be tonified. I have had nothing but bad results when I used a dispersing technique.

Another part of the treatment is lifestyle and dietary in nature. The choice of a lifestyle—a life that will help to build up the patient's energy—seems obvious. The diet is not quite so obvious. Many patients respond well to a gluten-free diet and to the addition of dietary supplements, including an increased amount of omega-3 fatty acids. Gluten is found in many grains, including wheat, and omega-3 fatty acids are found in flax seed oil, borage oil, and evening primrose oil.

Endnotes

1. Some of the suspected triggers for this condition include free radical damage, nutritional deficiency, increased blood vessel growth, poor circulation and shallow breathing, liver congestion, and a reduced amount of stomach acid. The elderly can certainly experience one or more of these adverse triggers.

2. Multiple sclerosis may be responsible for a full third of all cases.

3. This is an important cause of the illness in the elderly.

Chapter 8

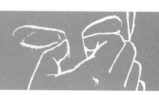

Fluid Problems

8.1 Glaucoma: An Introduction

Glaucoma is the name[1] given to an eye disease that is characterized by a loss of peripheral vision. Until recently, Western physicians believed that glaucoma was uniquely connected to abnormally elevated intraocular pressure. It has since been found that while most individuals with glaucoma have elevated intraocular pressure, approximately 25 to 40 percent of people with glaucoma have normal, not elevated, eye pressure, and at least half of those with elevated eye pressure never develop glaucoma. Thus, at present, there is no consensus as to whether glaucoma represents a state of elevated intraocular pressure (with or without blindness) or whether it represents a characteristic abnormal visual pattern (with or without raised pressure). Nevertheless, it is a dangerous disease in that it can lead to blindness. In its acute form, blindness can come very quickly. In the chronic forms, blindness comes more slowly, but it can easily creep up unnoticed.

Pathology

Most of the eyeball is very robust. The sclera is one of the toughest parts of the body and is very difficult to cut even with a surgeon's knife. Even the cornea is tough, and in most individuals, it can withstand high pressure. However, there is one weak spot at the back—the optic disc—where the optic nerve, the arteries, and the veins enter the eye. By its very nature, this point is structurally unsound. Of necessity, it has to be slightly flexible to accommodate movements of the eye, and it is this point that starts to deform when the intraocular pressure increases. With the aid of an ophthalmoscope, this is seen as a deeper-than-normal cavity. As the depth of the cavity increases, the optic nerve has to stretch to accommodate the change. The resultant stress on the optic nerve may then lead to significant symptoms, the most likely being a loss of peripheral vision. In extreme cases, there may be tunnel vision, but a pattern of blindness of the kind shown in Fig. 8.1 is more common.

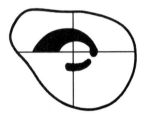

Fig. 8.1 Blindness pattern characteristic of glaucoma

Measurement of pressure in the eye

The normal pressure in the eye is about 13 to 15mmHg (approximately 25 mbar). This amount of pressure is quite low, equivalent to what you would find at the bottom of a pint jar. This pressure is enough to keep the eyeball 'inflated.' Under pathological conditions, the pressure can increase drastically to as much as 75mmHg, some five times the normal value. Individuals are said to have glaucoma if their intraocular pressure rises to 25mmHg, but some glaucoma symptoms have been reported at pressures as low as 19mmHg. This apparent paradox can be explained in traditional Chinese medicine (see below).

The old-fashioned way of measuring eye pressure was for the doctor to press on the eyeball to feel how hard it was, much in the same way as feeling the pressure in a bicycle tire. An improvement on that, but still old-fashioned, is a mechanical probe connected to a spring balance—an applanation tonometer—to measure the response of the eye. The optician will normally anesthetize the eye before doing the measurement. This is still in use in many places. More modern procedures include the use of an air-puff tonometer that uses a puff of air directed at the eyeball, rather than a mechanical probe. This is less invasive and does not require the eye to be anesthetized.

Types of glaucoma

The real problem with trying to classify glaucoma is that this disease is still not well understood by many practitioners. In older days, the disease was classified as either acute or chronic. Today this has been replaced by two other classifications that are based on the etiology of the disease:

- *Closed-angle (angle-closure) glaucoma.* This comprises almost 50 percent of the disease worldwide, but it is the less frequent type in the United States and Europe. It is usually acute when it represents a true emergency in that blindness can occur rapidly after the onset of symptoms. Acute closed-angle glaucoma is discussed in Section 8.2.

- *Chronic open-angle (chronic simple) glaucoma.* This is the most common type in the United States and Europe and is discussed in Section 8.3.

The difficulties in classifying and explaining the apparently conflicting symptoms can be explained in terms of traditional Chinese medicine. From a TCM point of view, there is a similarity between glaucoma and sciatica. In both, there may be a condition of excess or deficiency. Moreover, in both conditions, there may be significant physical distortions without any symptoms, or significant symptoms without noticeable physical distortions. In sciatica the patient may experience tingling sensations down the leg, pain, or numbness, all of which have their optical equivalents. Tingling would correspond to the visual disturbances such as seeing sparks of light or rainbow-like colors. Pain is simply pain where the whole eyeball may be intensely painful, or there may be referred pain in the head. Numbness would correspond to partial blindness. The acupuncturist should therefore treat the patient according to their pattern, as described below.

8.2   Acute Closed-Angle Glaucoma

Etiology

In closed-angle glaucoma, the pressure rises because the conduits for draining fluid from the eye become blocked while fluid keeps on pouring in. The blockage occurs when the iris curves forward and blocks the entrance to the drainage ducts known as Schlemm's canal (Fig. 8.2). In the majority of cases,[2] the pressure suddenly increases to high values (sometimes within a few hours). Thus, the primary cause of closed-angle glaucoma is simply mechanical closure. It is like putting a plug in a basin while the tap is running.

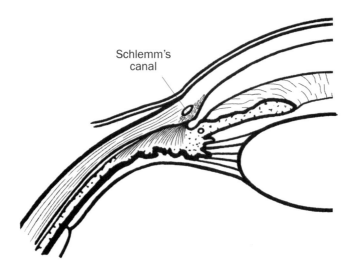

Schlemm's
canal

Fig. 8.2   Front of the eye and Schlemm's canal

In Western medicine the main external cause is considered to be stress and anxiety. There is also an internal contributing factor: an enlarged pupil.[3] The size of the pupil is controlled by the level of tension in the iris, a very thin piece of quite floppy flesh. The level of tension in the iris is controlled by two muscles: the sphincter muscle at the center, which is responsible for reducing the size of the aperture, and the dilator muscle, which covers most of the area of the iris (Fig. 8.3). The iris is held in tension, like a drum skin, by the opposition of these two muscles.

It is not entirely clear why the iris should deform enough to close the exit angle. One would expect the general level of tension that is present in the individual to spread to the eyes, making the muscles of the iris tense as well. In such circumstances, the iris would stretch tightly and not collapse.

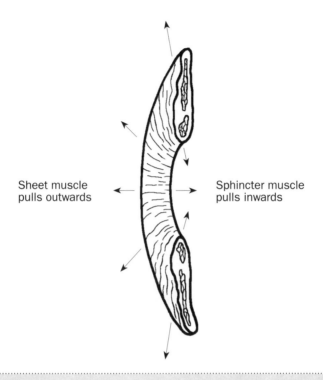

Sheet muscle
pulls outwards

Sphincter muscle
pulls inwards

Fig. 8.3 Muscles that control the iris

TCM approach

THREE MAIN PATTERNS

The three main patterns described in the Chinese texts are:

- Liver yang rising
- Kidney weakness
- Heart panic

The causes of the first two are straightforward. Liver yang rising is typically caused by repressed anger, while Kidney deficiency is caused by overwork and exhaustion. The third pattern, Heart panic, does not need much explanation as such—the cause is simply panic. What is slightly surprising is its inclusion as a pattern in-and-of-itself. It is recognized that a person need not be drastically ill to get acute glaucoma; they just have to be in an enormous state of anxiety. This pattern has also been recognized by Western medical physicians.

ANOTHER PATTERN SEEN IN WESTERN PATIENTS

The patterns for patients in the West are slightly different from those commonly seen in China. In the West, it is relatively uncommon to see full-blown cases of Liver yang rising with, for example, red face, red tongue and yellow coating, wiry pulse, and hypochondriac pain. It is more common in the West to see patients in a state of tension from too much mental work, especially from the tension and strain caused by spending too much time looking at computer screens, and from the stagnation brought about by cold and dampness. In place of volcanic anger, the Western patient is more likely to suffer from smoldering resentment. This combination of causes leads to a quite distinct pattern, which may be summed up by the term nervous excitability.

In clinical practice, this pattern is one of deficiency-stagnation, and although it appears quite differently from the Heart panic pattern, it may be treated in the same way.

SIGNS AND SYMPTOMS

▶ *General*
- headaches or eye pain in the affected eye[4]
- sensation of pressure in the eye
- visual disturbances (halos, sparks, and/or blind spots)
- difficulty in focusing
- possible nausea and vomiting

▶ *According to the Pattern*

Pattern	Signs and Symptoms
Liver yang rising	Red eyes Usually red face, although sometimes pale or green Frustration, tension, anger Occipital or temporal headache Wiry pulse Red or purple tongue
Kidney weakness	Headache is less severe or may occur on the weekends* Exhausted and overworked Weak or sore back Pulse weak, especially in the third position Tongue pale, possibly with red tip or red dots

Pattern	Signs and Symptoms
Heart panic	Face normally gray but may change History of stress Palpitations Insomnia
Nervous excitability	Thin Jumpy Pale face, perhaps a pasty look Poor appetite (may prefer to eat salads) Much mental stress Poor sleep

* It appears to be a characteristic of headaches from Kidney exhaustion that they are either dull or occur at times when the patient relaxes, typically on weekends. During the work week, one will exert one's willpower to maintain the circulation of qi and blood. One will 'keep oneself going' by the force of one's willpower.

TREATMENT

The proper place for a patient with acute closed-angle glaucoma is in the emergency room for the simple reason that if the elevated intraocular pressure continues for more than a few hours, there may be permanent damage to the eyesight. The back part of the eye will be so pushed out and distorted, and the optic nerve so stretched at that point, that the patient will go blind with little chance of recovery.

However, this does not mean that acupuncture should not be used. Quite the contrary! It should be the treatment of first choice in the emergency room. As anyone who has had acupuncture can testify, it has a marvelous relaxing effect. Problems in life that seemed huge before treatment no longer seem so great after the treatment. In addition, acupuncture has a great effect on each of the patterns. Furthermore, by using local and near points, qi can be brought to the eyes, which will have an immediate effect on the iris, and thus on intra-ocular pressure.

EMERGENCY TREATMENT

Three types of points that should be used, summarized in the following table.

Type of Point	Examples
Local* and near points	BL-1 (jing ming), ST-1 (cheng qi), M-HN-8 (qiu hou), GB-1 (tong zi liao), GB-20 (feng chi)
Calming points	LI-4 (he gu), LR-3 (tai chong), HT-7 (shen men)
Channel points that affect the eyes	BL-62 (shen mai), BL-63 (jin men), LR-2 (xing jian)

* See Fig. 5.2 for an illustration of how to needle these points.

▶ *Typical Emergency Room Prescription:*

BL-1 (jing ming)	LI-4 (he gu)
M-HN-8 (qiu hou)	LR-3 (tai chong)
GB-20 (feng chi)	

In case of panic, add:

HT-7 (shen men)	Calms the spirit
GV-19 (hou ding), GV-24 (shen ting), GB-13 (ben shen)	This combination has a powerful effect in calming panic

METHOD: The local points are stimulated so that a strong sensation is felt at first to release the qi stagnation. This is often likened to the sensation of an electrical shock. A few minutes later, the needles should be stimulated again to release further stagnation. When the associated tension has been relieved, a tonifying method may be used to bring the qi sensation to the back of the eye. This may involve the deep needling sensation described in Chapter 5.

GB-20 (feng chi) should be needled toward the opposite eye and, if possible, the sensation should reach the eye. LI-4 (he gu) and LR-3 (tai chong) should be needled with strong reducing technique. The remaining points should be needled with an even technique.

Follow-up treatment according to the pattern

The acupuncturist is more likely to see the patient after the visit to the emergency room, in which case the following treatments will be helpful. They may be used to supplement any Western medical treatment.

▶ *Liver Yang Rising*

TREATMENT PRINCIPLE: Bring qi to the eyes and calm the Liver qi.

BL-1 (*jing ming*)	Brings qi to the eyes
M-HN-8 (*qiu hou*)	Brings qi to the eyes
GB-20 (*feng chi*)	Brings qi to the eyes and calms the Liver qi
LI-4 (*he gu*) and LR-3 (*tai chong*)	Together they calm the Liver qi

METHOD: The tonifying method is used at points near the eyes while the dispersing method is used at the other points.

▶ *Kidney Weakness*

TREATMENT PRINCIPLE: Bring qi to the eyes and tonify the Liver and Kidneys.

BL-1 (*jing ming*)	Brings qi to the eyes
M-HN-8 (*qiu hou*)	Brings qi to the eyes
BL-18 (*gan shu*)	Strengthens the Liver and Kidneys
BL-23 (*shen shu*)	Strengthens the Liver and Kidneys
KI-3 (*tai xi*)	Strengthens the Kidneys

METHOD: The tonifying method is used at all the points.

▶ *Heart Panic and Nervous Excitability*

TREATMENT PRINCIPLE: Bring qi to the eyes and calm the spirit.

BL-1 (*jing ming*)	Brings qi to the eyes
M-HN-8 (*qiu hou*)	Brings qi to the eyes
GV-19 (*hou ding*), GV-24 (*shen ting*), and GB-13 (*ben shen*)	This combination has a powerful effect in calming panic
HT-7 (*shen men*)	Calms the spirit
PC-6 (*nei guan*)	Calms the spirit

METHOD: The tonifying method is used at points near the eyes while the even method is used at the other points. If the patient is thin and weak, either use moxibustion alone or combine moxibustion and needling at BL-23 *(shen shu)*.

Western medical and acupuncture treatment

Acute glaucoma must be treated urgently. In severe cases, total blindness can occur if the intraocular pressure remains very high for as little as 12 hours. In extreme cases like this, it is irresponsible to treat solely with acupuncture, and the proper place for the patient, as with any emergency, is in the emergency room. Typical Western medical treatment include:

- eye drops to constrict the iris, thereby pulling it away from the drainage channels
- medicines taken by mouth or intravenously to reduce intraocular pressure
- surgery—as a last resort—to create an artificial drainage channel

Western medicine has little in the way of long-term treatment to regulate the body condition so that this condition does not recur.

It is wonderful if the acupuncture can be performed in the emergency room. Emergency treatment is likely to have dramatic effects, and it is even possible that no medicine will need to be used. Once the emergency is over, acupuncture is of enormous benefit, for it can treat the underlying condition. This means that the patients can be weaned off their medications without danger of recurrence of the condition.

I have only treated a few cases of acute glaucoma. The effects were very striking, with the pain and sensation of pressure going down within hours of treatment. The symptoms returned a few days later, confirming the need for several treatments a week in the early stages.

Acupuncture treatment of the after-effects

The after-effect of acute glaucoma is likely to be partial blindness, which often has a characteristic shape (Fig. 8.1) as a result of the damage to the optic nerve. From the point of view of acupuncture, the treatments are the same as those given for any damaged nerve, such as numbness in the leg resulting from a damaged sciatic nerve. The following rules apply:

- *Intensive treatment is required.* The ideal is to give one treatment each day for 10 days, with a 4-day rest before resuming treatment. However, once a day for 5 days with a 2-day rest is a good second best. If the patient has only one treatment a week, it is unlikely that there will be much improvement. An alternative to daily acupuncture treatment is the home use of microcurrent electrical stimulation (see below).

- *Approximately 100 treatments are necessary.* The Chinese texts, as well as my own experience with Western patients, indicate that between 50 and 150 treatments may be required. To many acupuncturists, this may seem like an excessive number, but it would be misleading to suggest that fewer treatments will be sufficient. Moreover, if there is a chance of restoring the eyesight, the time and expense is well worth it.

- *Treatment is much more successful if begun within 3 months of the nerve injury.* If it is started more than 2 years after the injury, only minor changes are likely to occur.

TREATMENT

Frequent local stimulation, preferably reaching the optic nerve, is the number one aim of treatment. The details of treatment may be left to the practitioner. Below we give a typical prescription of points that may be used with the conventional acupuncture needle. The points round the eye may also be chosen for stimulation with a microcurrent electrical stimulator (see next page).

BL-1 (*jing ming*)	Brings qi to the eyes
M-HN-8 (*qiu hou*)	Brings qi to the eyes
GB-20 (*feng chi*)	Brings qi to the eyes
ST-36 (*zu san li*)	Tonifies the overall qi
LR-3 (*tai chong*)	Regulates the Liver and benefits the eyes

Alternatives to ST-36 and LR-3 include:

BL-20 (*pi shu*)	Strengthens the Spleen and Liver
BL-18 (*gan shu*)	Strengthens the Kidney and Liver
BL-23 (*shen shu*)	Strengthens the Kidney and Liver

METHOD: When needling the local points—BL-1 *(jing ming)*, ST-1 *(cheng qi)*, M-HN-8 *(qiu hou)*—the sensation should reach to the back of the eye. Ideally, this should be a warm, comfortable sensation. In the later stages of treatment, when the qi is flowing well, these points need only be needled to a depth of 0.5 unit to get the sensation to reach immediately to the back of the eye, but in the early stages of treatment, it may be necessary to needle to a heroic depth of 2 units before any sensation is felt at the back of the eye. (See Chapter 5 for further notes on needling these sensitive points.)

When needling near points, such as GB-20 *(feng chi)*, again, the ideal is to get the sensation to reach the eye, but treatment can often be effective in patients where you only manage to achieve local qi sensation. The distal points—ST-36 *(zu san li)*, LR-3 *(tai chong)*, BL-18 *(gan shu)*, BL-20 *(pi shu)*, BL-23 *(shen shu)*—are needled with the tonifying method.

RESULTS: If the rules described above are followed, there is a good chance that daytime eyesight will be completely restored. There may be some slight reduction of night vision in the affected areas.

MICROCURRENT ELECTRICAL STIMULATION

The microcurrent stimulator is of great benefit in treating the after effects of glaucoma. Patients can do the treatments themselves, up to three times a day, without the need of coming to the clinic. With this intensity of treatment, patients need only come to the clinic once or twice a week to regulate the overall qi.

8.3   Chronic Open-Angle Glaucoma

Etiology

The onset of open-angle glaucoma is more insidious. The pressure gradually creeps up,[5] and the retina and nerves gradually deaden, often without any pain or even discomfort. Gradually, blind areas appear at the edge of the field of vision. To the patient, they do not appear as black areas. Rather, the patient will have trouble differentiating between varying shades of light and dark. In addition, the eyes gradually become oversensitive to light, and night vision deteriorates. However, just as most people are unaware of their 'blind spot' (the point of the visual field that corresponds to the optic disc), many are unaware of the loss of sight from glaucoma until quite large areas of the visual field have been destroyed, by which time it may be too late to do anything.

TCM approach

In the past in China, there were no instruments for measuring the pressure inside the eyes so glaucoma as a diagnosis was unknown. The symptoms of glaucoma were well explained in terms of a slow onset of blindness. It is only recently, with the development of combined TCM and Western medical eye clinics, that the differentiation has been worked out.

Some books give a slightly different list of patterns for glaucoma and for other degenerative diseases of the eye, but others simply group together the diseases of glaucoma, macular degeneration, and optic atrophy (including retinitis pigmentosa). It is the latter approach that we have taken here, for it seems much more straightforward. Interestingly, something of this approach can be seen lurking beneath the surface of Western medicine since clinicians are starting to realize that elevated intraocular pressure does not necessarily lead to visual impairment, and, conversely, the loss of peripheral vision so characteristic of glaucoma can happen at very low pressure. It is recognized that people can sustain pressures of 30mmHg (40mbar) for long periods of time without sustaining any damage to their eyes. It is obvious, therefore, that there is more to the question than just the intraocular pressure.

A further cause that must be considered is mercury leaching out of dental fillings. This can gradually seep up toward the eyes and can interfere with the proper circulation of fluids in the nose and eyes. Western medicine recognizes the effect of other chemicals such as lead and methanol as causative agents for optic neuritis. Perhaps one day the role of mercury in these degenerative disorders will be addressed. (See Section 4.4 and Appendix 3 for a fuller discussion of the effects of mercury.)

CAUSES OF ELEVATED INTRAOCULAR PRESSURE

A more complete explanation of how the eyesight becomes injured is given in Section 8.1, but it is worth spending a little time here on the related topic of elevated eye pressure. As mentioned earlier, the patterns associated with increased intraocular pressure are:

- Liver yang rising
- Kidney weakness
- Spleen qi deficiency
- Lung qi deficiency

These are the same patterns that are given in many Chinese books for high blood pressure, and they need only be modified slightly for Western patients. Looked at from this simple point of view, the etiology and pathology of the patterns can be discerned.

▶ *Liver Yang Rising*

The energy rises up to the eye, and, as it rises, it carries fluids with it.[6] The result is increased flow *into* the eye. If this is not compensated for by increased outflow, then the internal eye pressure will increase. The underlying condition of Liver yang rising is usually the result of frustration and anger combined with a sedentary life and rich food. In some patients it is the result of a very stressful job. The signs and symptoms are:

- patient is under stress
- frequently has strong headaches
- pale or purplish face
- purple tongue
- wiry pulse

Western patients tend to suffer more from long periods of frustration and resentment than from full-blown anger. In younger people this may show as a red face with a green color around the mouth (women) or bluish color around the mouth and the cheeks (men). In older people it manifests as an overall red face with a sort of 'turkey crop' fold hanging between the chin and throat. The predominant energy coming from these people is that of irritability rather than pure anger.

▶ *Kidney Weakness*

This pattern is listed as Kidney yin deficiency in some books, but I prefer the term Kidney weakness *(xū ruò)* given in other books because usually both the Kidney yin and yang are weakened. In this pattern, the flow of fluids *out* of the eye is reduced because the Kidneys are not properly performing their function of controlling the fluids. The underlying condition of Kidney weakness occurs naturally in old age. It may also appear in patients who have abused their bodies with a reckless lifestyle, including the use of drugs. This condition may also occur during menopause, especially when there is mercury in the system (see Appendix 3). The signs and symptoms are:

- patient looks old or tired
- hair is thinning
- facial color may be pale or bright red
- sore or weak back
- arthritis
- pulse may be weak but more often is long, characteristic of hardening of the arteries

▶ *Spleen Qi Deficiency*

This pattern is often described as Spleen and Kidney yang deficiency, and frequently the Kidneys are also involved, certainly in cases where the sight is impaired. However, the essential imbalance here is in the composition of fluids in the eyes. Instead of being a clear fluid, the aqueous humor becomes turbid (or thick) and viscous, so that it does not flow easily through the very fine network of the trabeculae (see Chapter 1). The underlying condition is usually said to be the result of hard work, irregular meals, and being overtired. It is a common pattern among working mothers. The signs and symptoms are:

- gray face
- tendency to being overweight
- digestion feels uncomfortable, regardless of the diet
- may overeat
- pale tongue, possibly coated (perhaps with stringy saliva)
- slippery pulse

In the West the conventional pattern is sometimes seen, but, more commonly, the problem results from an accumulation of phlegm. The Spleen may indeed show signs of weakness, but the root cause is not so much hard work weakening the Spleen. Rather, it is an accumulation of cold and dampness from cold and damp food and medicines, which has led to the formation of phlegm.

▶ *Lung Qi Deficiency*

The Lungs rule the descending and dispersing of fluids. Therefore, any fluids that accumulate in the head are likely to be due to an obstruction of Lung qi. This pattern is not given in every book. The signs and symptoms are:

- pale or white face
- quiet voice

- may have history of asthma or other Lung illness
- possibly has frequent infections
- often a dip or discoloration in the Lung area of the tongue
- may have 'bean-bone'[7] pulse

In the West, straightforward Lung qi deficiency is not seen that often because lung infections are quickly treated with antibiotics and also because the sort of hard physical labor that injures the lungs is uncommon. More common is an obstruction to the flow of Lung qi. This may be a result of an incompletely cured pathogenic factor (as a result of antibiotic treatment), thick phlegm, or prolonged grief. Sometimes it is simply a lack of exercise. In some patients the Lung problem manifests as asthma.

TREATMENT

It is well worth matching the treatment to the main presenting pattern of the patient. I would like to draw the reader's attention to the choice of points for the Spleen qi deficiency and Lung qi deficiency patterns. LR-3 is not used to treat these patterns, even though this point is considered the number one point for the eyes. In the other two patterns—Liver yang rising and Kidney weakness—this point may be used, but other points may be found to be better. As a general principle of treatment, local and near points are used to bring qi to the eyes while distal points are used to treat the underlying energetic imbalance. Both local and near points as well as pattern-specific points are shown below.

▶ *Local and Near Points*

In all treatments, points will be needed to bring qi to the eyes. Such points include:

BL-1 *(jing ming)*
ST-1 *(cheng qi)*
GB-20 *(feng chi)*

METHOD: The points near the eyes only need to be needled to a medium depth. When manipulating these points, a warm sensation should fill the eyes.

▶ *Liver Yang Rising*

TREATMENT PRINCIPLE: Bring qi to the eyes and calm the Liver yang.
In addition to the main points, add:

LR-3 (*tai chong*)	Calms the Liver yang
LR-2 (*xing jian*)	Calms the Liver fire
LI-4 (*he gu*)	Calms the Liver yang when combined with LR-3 (*tai chong*)

METHOD: The dispersing method is used at all the points.

▶ *Kidney Weakness*

TREATMENT PRINCIPLE: Bring qi to the eyes and strengthen the Kidneys.
In addition to the main points, add:

KI-3 (*tai xi*)	Tonifies the Kidneys
BL-23 (*shen shu*)	Tonifies the Kidneys
LR-3 (*tai chong*)	Tonifies the Liver and brightens the eyes
BL-18 (*gan shu*)	Tonifies the Liver

METHOD: These points are tonified; the back associated points may be treated with moxibustion as well as needled.

▶ *Spleen Qi Deficiency*

TREATMENT PRINCIPLE: Bring qi to the eyes and tonify the Spleen.
In addition to the main points, add:

SI-6 (*yang lao*)	Brightens the eyes
ST-36 (*zu san li*)	Tonifies the Stomach, Spleen, and Kidneys
SP-6 (*san yin jiao*)	Tonifies Spleen, Liver and Kidneys
CV-12 (*zhong wan*)	Front *mu* point of the Spleen

METHOD: All these points are tonified. Needling may be followed by moxibustion. If there is much mucus, use the even technique at ST-40 (*feng long*) with no moxibustion.

▶ *Lung Qi Deficiency*

TREATMENT PRINCIPLE: Bring qi to the eyes and tonify the Lung qi.
In addition to the main points, add:

LU-7 (*lie que*)	Benefits the Lungs
LU-9 (*tai yuan*)	Tonifies the Lung qi
BL-13 (*fei shu*)	Tonifies the Lungs; back associated (*shu*) point of the Lungs

METHOD: All the points are tonified. Moxibustion may be used at BL-13 *(fei shu)*.

FREQUENCY OF TREATMENT

At first, treatment should be given three times a week. If given only once a week, the outcome is uncertain. After the initial stage, treatment may be reduced to once a week.

RESULTS

There should be no difficulty in bringing down the pressure in the eyes and relieving the symptoms of glaucoma as long as the patient comes for treatment. It is difficult to describe the long-term effects with any degree of accuracy because the range of patients and the range of conditions vary widely. If the patient has a clear pattern with many of the signs and symptoms fitting together appropriately, then the prognosis is more favorable. As with high blood pressure, some patients are completely cured, while others (particularly the elderly) require regular booster treatments. This may be another area where the microcurrent electrical stimulator will be of great use.

Western medical and acupuncture treatment

Strangely, the Western medical treatment for open-angle glaucoma is the same as for closed-angle glaucoma. The same eye drops are put into the eye: medicines that have the effect of contracting the ciliary muscle and of reducing the aperture of the pupil. Apparently, the precise mechanism by which the medication works is not fully understood. The treatment is simple and relatively non-invasive. The main disadvantage is that it must be done every single day. There is also a less publicized disadvantage: a slightly increased risk of heart failure among patients who use these drops regularly.

There are other local treatments that are used to reduce the aqueous secretion into the eyes. One of these is digoxin, the drug from foxglove, *Digitalis spp.*, which benefits the heart.

The role of acupuncture here is similar to its role in the management of high blood pressure. When the condition arises from old age, acupuncture can be of great benefit, but there is little chance of a complete cure. This means that once the pressure in the eyes has been brought down to reasonable levels, the patient must come regularly for maintenance treatments, say every three to four weeks. Not all patients will do this, and many prefer to take eye drops. If the patient is younger, then by changing the body condition, there is hope of a complete cure.

Still, whatever the age of the patient, acupuncture *is of benefit*. However, it must be stressed that any reduction in the intake of drugs should be done in conjunction with an ophthalmologist or optometrist so that regular checks on the eye pressure can be made.

8.4 Watering Eyes

TCM approach

THUMBNAIL SKETCH OF THE PATTERNS

This is perhaps the most common eye problem seen by acupuncturists. As would be expected of a common symptom, there are many different underlying patterns, both in Western and Chinese medicine. From the point of view of Western medicine, this would cover a range of conditions from conjunctivitis to hay fever to 'idiopathic' watering eyes.

In terms of Chinese medicine, the common patterns are:

- wind-heat
- Liver qi stagnation
- lingering pathogenic factor*
- Lung and Spleen qi deficiency*
- Heart fire
- Bladder channel damp-heat
- Blood insufficiency
- Liver and Kidney weakness

These are the patterns commonly given in the Chinese texts devoted to oph-thalmology, except for those marked with an asterisk, which derive from my own clinical experience with Western patients. By contrast, general acupuncture textbooks may give no differentiation at all, or, more commonly, the material is divided into 'hot tears' and 'cold tears'. This is the differentiation given in *Essential Subtleties on the Silver Sea (Yin hai jing wei)* and is based on a differentiation between a condition of excess, usually Liver heat, and a condition of deficiency, usually Liver and Kidney weakness. A key differentiating symptom is that hot tears flow when facing away from the wind, and cold tears flow when facing into the wind.

Briefly, the eight patterns can be summarized as follows:

Wind-heat	Infection of the eye, 'pink eye,' or conjunctivitis. Sudden onset (within a day).
Liver qi stagnation	Many chronic conditions, including hay fever and watering eyes when going outside. Generally, the patients are fairly strong but tense.
Lingering pathogenic factor	Hay fever, which is often a pattern that started in childhood. The pathogenic factor lies dormant in the eyes and nose and is 'awoken' at the onset of spring or in response to an allergen.
Lung and Spleen qi deficiency	May have seasonal watering eyes, such as hay fever or autumnal allergy to molds, or may just have watering eyes when tired or upset.
Heart fire	Red faced, jolly types. "I laughed until the tears ran down my face."
Blood insufficiency	Eyes often feel dry and gritty even though they are watering.
Liver and Kidney weakness	Seen in older patients and women at menopause. Patients feel tired and lack enthusiasm for life.
Bladder channel damp-heat	An all-purpose, catch-all pattern for everything else! Often associated with stiff back, maybe slight urinary problems, and headache in the occiput.

TEARS AND THE FIVE YIN ORGANS

Tears are the body fluid associated with the phase wood, since the eyes pertain to the Liver and the Liver pertains to wood. In clinical practice, while this is often true, it is by no means always the case.

Looked at from the point of view of TCM, there are three main organs responsible for body fluids, including the production of tears: Lungs, Spleen, and

Kidneys. An imbalance in any one of these can allow dampness to accumulate, which may manifest as tears. However, the Lungs are the most important of the three since the Lungs relate to fluid imbalances in the upper part of the body.

BLOOD INSUFFICIENCY

As first sight, it is surprising that blood insufficiency would cause excessive production of tears. Rather, dry eyes would be expected, to be consistent with the general dry nature of blood insufficiency. The reason this condition produces wet eyes rather than dry eyes can be deduced from an understanding of the physiology of the tear ducts.

There are two types of glands in the eyelid: those found all over the inner surface of the eyelid that carry the normal tear secretion, and those specialized ones that are distributed on the margin of the eyelid that carry the oily secretion known as meibomium. Because of its oily nature, the meibomium reduces the surface tension of the tear film and prevents it from breaking up. Since blood insufficiency is characterized by, among other things, dryness and lack of lubricating oil, the eye is not lubricated by oil or by tears. As a consequence, the eye gets very irritated. It is the irritation that leads to ever more production of tears.[8]

Etiology and pathology

▶ *Wind-Heat*

This pattern arises simply because of an attack of wind. In terms of Western medicine, the wind-heat pattern is very close to conjunctivitis, which is thought to be brought on by a bacterial infection. Usually, underlying the infection there is heat, either from unsuitable food (e.g., highly processed food containing large amounts of additives), or from a change in the weather from cold to warm. The signs and symptoms are:

- red, sore, and watering eyes, possibly with purulent discharge
- patient is quite strong
- sudden onset
- rapid, full, and floating pulse

▶ *Liver Qi Stagnation*

The cause of this pattern given in the Chinese texts is 'restraint of the seven emotions,' which usually means the restraint of anger. The anger can generally be related to an obvious external cause. In the West we have more opportunity to vent our anger and to answer back, so this is not such a common cause. More common here is a general state of being angry, where the underlying anger does not find expression or may even not be recognized as such. The origin of this may well be a lingering pathogenic factor, as described below. Over a period of time, a feeling of rage leads to stagnation of Liver qi and then to Liver heat. Signs and symptoms are:

- eyes water in the wind
- may appear to be very angry or tense, but more often has irritability alternating with great charm
- tendency to high blood pressure
- red tongue
- wiry pulse

▶ *Lingering Pathogenic Factor*

A lingering pathogenic factor is an imbalance resulting from an invasion of a pathogenic factor that is never quite resolved. The patient never quite recovers from an illness, and there is something remaining of the original pathogenic factor. If it was hot, as is often the case with infections, then there may be heat lingering in the body. This pattern often starts early in childhood. It is commonly seen in cases of myalgic encephalomyelitis and in glandular fever, a term used to describe such diverse illnesses as mononucleosis and fibromyalgia. The origin of lingering pathogenic factors is described in more detail in *Acupuncture in the Treatment of Children* (3rd ed., p. 43). The signs and symptoms are:

- symptom is seasonal, often in the springtime
- although spring is the worst time, the patient does not seem to be very angry
- often has a history of Lung problems
- may have signs of thick phlegm
- slippery, rather than wiry, pulse

▶ *Lung and Spleen Qi Deficiency*

In principle this pattern can arise from overwork, but the type of overwork that causes the pattern is hard physical labor. It is now rare in the West for there are not many people who have to do grueling physical work. A more common pattern now is lack of sleep, especially during the formative years of childhood.

It is quite likely that these patients have a history of asthma. Signs and symptoms are:

- pale face
- quiet voice
- poor appetite or excessive eating
- thin and lacking in energy or overweight
- frequent infections
- possibly has history of asthma
- weak pulse

Additionally, these patients may have the following symptoms characteristic of mucous conditions:

- nasal discharge
- cough
- slippery pulse

▶ *Heart Fire*

This pattern generally refers simply to excess heat in the body that then affects the Heart. Its most common cause is eating the types of food that create excess heat, such as spicy foods and alcohol. Signs and symptoms include:

- face red
- eyes red
- inner canthus is especially red, inflamed, and painful
- restlessness
- insomnia
- tongue red with thick yellow coating
- rapid and slippery pulse

▶ *Bladder Channel Damp-Heat*

This pattern is a general catch-all. Common causes are overexposure to damp weather, eating too many dampness-producing foods, or mercury building up in the body. Signs and symptoms include:

- stiff back
- may have slight urinary problems
- may have to urinate more than once at a time
- ache in the occiput

▶ *Blood Insufficiency*

Common causes of blood insufficiency are blood loss as a result of, for example, heavy periods or difficult childbirth, and insufficient iron intake to compensate for this loss of blood. The life situation that encourages this pattern is one where the will becomes completely subdued. For example, it can happen when a woman has a dominating and controlling partner. It is particularly common among women who are stuck at home with very young children and are unable to do anything for themselves because of the constant demands of the children. Signs and symptoms include:

- face gray
- dry or brittle hair
- tired
- lives off nervous energy
- pale tongue

▶ *Liver and Kidney Weakness*

There are various causes for this pattern, the most common of which is overwork. In China, overwork usually means physical overwork, but this pattern can arise from any sort of overwork, especially when it is combined with irregular working hours. Other causes are simply old age and the changes that women go through at menopause. These can be especially difficult and are particularly likely to give rise to watering eyes if there is a large amount of mercury in the system. Signs and symptoms include:

- sore back
- weak knees
- arthritis
- poor memory
- low vitality
- no interest in life

TREATMENT

▶ *Local and Near Points*

In all the treatments, local and near points are used to bring qi to the eyes, for example:

BL-1 *(jing ming)*, ST-1 *(cheng qi)*, or GB-20 *(feng chi)*

The points near the eyes need only be needled quite superficially so that the qi sensation goes to the front of the eyes. In conditions of excess, the sensation may be quite strong as the excess qi is dispersed, while in deficiency, the sensation is milder, as is normal with tonifying. In treating hot disorders, there may be a cool sensation coming from the needles.

▶ *Wind-Heat*

TREATMENT PRINCIPLE: Clear and cool the wind-heat.
The distal point GB-20 *(feng chi)* listed above is an important point for this pattern since it clears wind and heat as well as brightens the eyes. In addition to the use of this point and BL-1 and ST-1, add:

LI-4 *(he gu)*	Clears wind and brings qi to the eyes (via the channel)
GB-37 *(guang ming)*	Benefits the eyes and clears heat

If there is obvious dampness and discharge in the eye, add:

GB-34 *(yang ling quan)*	Clears phlegm-dampness from the Liver and Gallbladder

Other useful points include:

GV-23 *(shang xing)*	Brings qi to the eyes
TB-3 *(zhong zhu)*	Very good for mild attacks of conjunctivitis; it has the advantage of not interfering too much with the patient's qi circulation

METHOD: Use the reducing method at all the points.

▶ *Liver Qi Stagnation*

TREATMENT PRINCIPLE: Move the Liver qi.
In addition to the main points, add:

LI-4 *(he gu)* and LR-3 *(tai chong)*	Pair strongly moves the Liver qi
GB-37 *(guang ming)*	Moves the Liver qi and benefits the eyes

METHOD: The even or dispersing method is used.

RESULTS: If the problem is of relatively recent onset and the cause of the strong anger is clearly understood, the treatment will likely be effective. However, more often the pattern has been present since childhood and only after many years of incubation has it finally manifested as watering eyes. For patients like this, the treatment will be surprisingly successful in the short term, with striking results after about five treatments, but there is the likelihood that they must keep coming back for treatment, especially at times of external stress.

▶ *Lingering Pathogenic Factor*

TREATMENT PRINCIPLE: Bring qi to the eyes, clear the lingering pathogenic factor, and improve the circulation of qi.
In addition to the main points, add:

M-HN-30 (*bai lao*)	Clears lingering pathogenic factors
BL-18 (*gan shu*)	Softens thick phlegm and clears lingering pathogenic factors
BL-20 (*pi shu*)	Softens thick phlegm and clears lingering pathogenic factors

METHOD: The even or moving method is used at all these points.

RESULTS: If the problem is of recent onset, there is a good possibility of clearing it altogether in about 10 treatments. Much more likely is that the patient has myalgic encephalomyelitis or fibromyalgia, and the pattern is deeply rooted in the body. In such cases, treatment can help to control the symptom of watering eyes, but it is unlikely to provide a lasting cure until the underlying pattern is finally eliminated.

▶ *Lung and Spleen Qi Deficiency*

TREATMENT PRINCIPLE: Bring qi to the eyes and tonify the Lung and Spleen qi.
In addition to the main points, add:

LU-9 (*tai yuan*)	Tonifies the Lung qi
BL-13 (*fei shu*)	Tonifies the Lungs (back associated [*shu*] point of Lungs)
ST-36 (*zu san li*)	Tonifies the Stomach and Spleen
SP-6 (*san yin jiao*)	Tonifies the Spleen, Kidneys, and Liver
BL-20 (*pi shu*)	Tonifies the Spleen and Liver (back associated [*shu*] point of Spleen)

METHOD: The tonifying method is used at all the points.

RESULTS: If the pattern is of recent onset, especially if it follows a particularly exhausting time, 5 to 10 treatments may well cure the problem completely. Much more likely is that the watering eyes are the result of a pattern that endured since early childhood, in which case it is very difficult to clear out altogether.

▶ *Heart Fire*

TREATMENT PRINCIPLE: Clear heat from the eyes and clear Heart fire.

The distal point GB-20 *(feng chi)* is an important one for this pattern since it clears heat as well as brightens the eyes. In addition to this point, BL-1 *(jing ming)*, and ST-1 *(cheng qi)*, add:

HT-8 *(shao fu)*	Clears Heart fire
LR-2 *(xing jian)*	Clears Liver fire and brightens the eyes

METHOD: The dispersing method is used at all points.

An alternative treatment is to bleed M-HN-10 *(er jian)*.

▶ *Bladder Channel Damp-Heat*

TREATMENT PRINCIPLE: Circulate qi in the eyes and clear damp-heat.

In addition to the main points, add:

BL-60 *(kun lun)*	Circulates the qi in the Bladder channel
BL-67 *(zhi yin)*	Clears heat from the Bladder channel and benefits the eyes

METHOD: The even or dispersing method is used. If the qi in the eyes is very congested, more dispersing is used.

▶ *Blood Insufficiency*

TREATMENT PRINCIPLE: Bring qi to the eyes and strengthen the blood.

In addition to the main points, add:

ST-36 *(zu san li)*	Tonifies the Spleen to generate blood
SP-6 *(san yin jiao)*	Tonifies the Spleen to generate blood
LR-8 *(qu quan)*	Strengthens Liver blood

METHOD: The tonifying method is used at all the points. (See Appendix 2 for a fuller discussion of this pattern.) If the patient is still losing a large amount of blood (e.g., from heavy periods), this should be addressed as a priority. Typical treatments for this are given in general acupuncture textbooks. If there is significant blood loss, acupuncture on its own may not be enough. This is one of the situations where herbal medicine can be more effective. If it is available, the patent medicine Eight-Treasure Decoction (*ba zhen tang*), also known as Women's Precious Pill, will be helpful. In addition, the patient will also benefit from mineral and vitamin supplements.

RESULTS: The results of acupuncture are variable. If the origin of the problem is more physical, then treatment will be more effective, while if the origin is more mental and emotional, the results are unpredictable. Sometimes the treatments are enough to turn a person's life around completely so that the individual never suffers from the pattern again. In other patients, acupuncture treatment is almost ineffective. And in still others, herbal prescriptions are effective, but they must be continued. The moment that they stop, the problems will return until some significant change takes place in the patient's life, such as the children growing up.

▶ *Liver and Kidney Weakness*

TREATMENT PRINCIPLE: Bring qi to the eyes and strengthen the Liver and Kidneys.

BL-18 (*gan shu*)	Tonifies the Liver and Kidneys
BL-20 (*pi shu*)	Tonifies the Spleen and Liver
BL-23 (*shen shu*)	Tonifies the Liver and Kidneys

METHOD: The tonifying method is used, usually with moxibustion as well as needles.

RESULTS: If the patient is still young, there is a good chance of curing the problem completely. The same is true of women at menopause. Typically 10 to 20 treatments are needed. Progress can be slow at first, and patients do get discouraged. However, the practitioner will notice a steady improvement. If the patient is very old, results are likely to be slow and doubtful.

Addendum: blocked tear ducts

Watering eyes is a symptom of blocked tear ducts and, as such, is covered by the descriptions given in this chapter. However, since it has such a specific diagnosis in terms of Western medicine, some comment is in order.

For a diagnosis of blocked tear duct, there must be something blocking the duct, and that something is mucus. This can arise from several sources. It could be an excess of heat, causing local inflammation and a corresponding buildup of mucus. It could come from general accumulation of phlegm in the system, so that the blocked tear duct is just one of many orifices that gets blocked from time to time. It could come from qi deficiency when there is insufficient qi to clear the mucus that has accumulated after a cold in the head. With this background, we can turn to the patterns that are likely to result in a blocked tear duct. The patterns related to heat are:

- Liver qi stagnation
- Heart fire

The patterns related to phlegm in the system are:

- lingering pathogenic factor
- Bladder channel damp-heat

The deficiency patterns are:

- Lung and Spleen qi deficiency
- Liver and Kidney weakness

Author's experience

My experience in treating blocked tear ducts is exclusively with children under the age of 14 years. In this age group, there are just two patterns that I have seen:

- lingering pathogenic factor
- Lung and Spleen weakness

Both of these patterns respond very well to acupuncture treatment.

Endnotes

1. The word 'glaucoma' is derived from the ancient Greek word *glaucos* (γλαυκυς), which referred to a blue-green hue found in a variety of eye illnesses, including the one we now call glaucoma. It is interesting to note that in Chinese, glaucoma is called *qīng máng* (blue-green blindness).

2. As noted above, a small percentage of patients develop a chronic form of this condition.

3. Factors that can cause the pupils to dilate are darkness or dim light, stress or excitement, and certain medications such as antihistamines, antidepressants, and eye drops used to dilate the pupils.

4. Acute closed-angle glaucoma usually affects one eye at a time, but the other eye is at risk of an attack as well.

5. While in closed-angle glaucoma the drainage angle formed by the cornea and iris closes or becomes blocked (see Section 8.2 and Fig. 8.2), in open-angle glaucoma the drainage angle remains open. Nevertheless, the aqueous humor drains too slowly, leading to fluid backup and the buildup of pressure in the eyes.

6. This is also observed in some cases of high blood pressure, watering eyes, and nasal discharge.

7. A bean-bone pulse is one that can be felt on the radial artery just distal to the wrist line. In a healthy person it should not be possible to feel this pulse. Its presence indicates injury to the lung organ, for example, by whooping cough when the individual was young or tuberculosis.

8. This is known in Western medicine as the 'foreign body response.' In a healthy eye, it has the function of washing out any foreign bodies and dust.

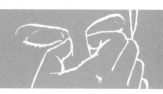

Chapter 9

Lens Problems

9.1 Cataract

Cataract is a common disease of old age. There are few people over the age of 60 who do not have the beginning of a cataract. In most people the cataract never develops far and may be little more than a small 'milky' dot in part of the lens (Fig. 9.1). In others, this milkiness can, but not necessarily will, extend to the whole lens, with the opacity gradually becoming worse until the lens resembles a hard boiled egg.[1]

In the early stages a cataract often starts as a localized cloudy area. At first, there may be just one or two diffuse spots that may well be off-center, and so the vision may be unaffected except in poor light when the pupil is fully dilated. Gradually, these spots grow in size and in opacity. Patients initially may be unaware of a cataract developing. Then they may perceive halos around objects, or things may become blurred. Gradually the vision deteriorates such that it is more and more difficult to read and to discern objects. In addition, patients can develop a so-called 'second sight' whereby, for a short interval, the eyesight actually appears to improve. This second sight does not last.

The treatment of cataract has become so much the province of the specialist eye surgeon that it may be forgotten that there are indeed other ways of treating it, with acupuncture being one and herbs and homeopathy being two others.

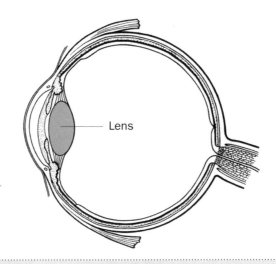

Fig. 9.1 The lens

The success of acupuncture in treating cataracts is not so well documented, but there are some impressive results in the Chinese literature about the effects of herbal treatments.

Etiology

FREE RADICALS

The lens gradually becomes more opaque as the proteins that form the lens degrade. This process occurs naturally with time and is somewhat analogous to the degradation of plastics in sunlight. It is thought that the process is accelerated by the presence of free radicals in the blood. These can come from many causes, including the imperfect digestion of meat and other proteins and insufficient levels of vegetables. Another cause are food items that contain free radicals or that are likely to promote the formation of free radicals. This includes most factory-produced foods and many vegetable fats, including sunflower oil, canola oil, and margarine. Other causes include the ultraviolet light in sunlight, cigarette smoke (which is rich in free radicals and toxins), photosensitizing drugs (such as some gout medications, cholesterol-lowering drugs, antibiotics, and diuretics), and steroid drugs (including corticosteroids, which are often prescribed by Western physicians for eye conditions).

From the point of view of Chinese medicine, these would all contribute to one or another of the patterns. Any of the patterns below could arise when there are excess free radicals.

DIABETES

Those who have diabetes are more likely to develop cataracts, although diabetes is usually associated in people's minds with retinopathy, rather than cataracts. The exact mechanism by which diabetes affects the lens is not known.

From the point of view of Chinese medicine, the cataract is probably not caused by the diabetes itself but by the imbalance that caused diabetes in the first place. This imbalance is essentially a product of heat consuming the yin of the Lungs, Spleen, and Kidneys. As can be seen from the list below, Kidney yin deficiency and Lung heat are among the patterns likely to lead to the formation of a cataract. Thus, to prevent or reverse the cataract, it is only necessary to cure the underlying imbalance, not to cure the diabetes, which is much harder.

TCM approach

ETIOLOGY AND PATHOLOGY

The lens is said to be kept clear and transparent by the body fluids. When the body fluids become 'turbid', cataracts will gradually develop. The body fluids are governed by the Kidneys and can become turbid when the Kidney yin is exhausted.

The prevalence of cataracts in old age is due to the gradual decline of Kidney yin with age. Imbalances that were small in youth become gradually bigger. Usually the imbalances that give rise to cataracts have been there for years and years, maybe since childhood. During childhood the imbalance was merely one of heat. In middle age there may have been minor problems, and then as old age creeps on, these imbalances start to cause real problems. Common among these problems is the onset of high blood pressure. Cataract is another one.

The Lungs are also responsible for the circulation of body fluids in that they condense the fluids sent up by the Kidneys. If the Lungs become dry or, worse still, if they become overheated, not enough fluid is condensed and returned to the Kidneys and that the fluids then become turbid.

External causes can include injury to the eye and excessive heat, especially infrared radiation, reaching the eye. This condition used to be a common affliction of welders and blacksmiths before heat-filtering glass was available.

Patterns	Signs and Symptoms
Liver and Kidney yin deficiency	Face or cheeks red, occasionally a pale face Weak or sore back Easily tired May have high blood pressure Red tongue
Lung dryness and Lung heat	Chronic Lung problems, such as chronic bronchitis or asthma Bean-bone pulse (see Section 8.3) Back bowed over in the thoracic area Dry skin

Liver and Kidney yin deficiency is by far the most common pattern, and there are many presentations. It occurs when there is simultaneously heat in the body and a gradual decline of Kidney energy. The heat may arise from many different causes, including Liver heat or Stomach heat. The gradual decline of Kidney energy may simply come from old age or from overwork. The variation in causes is reflected in the different facial colors. The most common is a red face with white over most of the rest of the body, as is often seen in older people with high blood pressure.[2] However, one also sees the characteristic red cheeks of yin deficiency as well as a pale or greenish face, which is characteristic of Liver stagnation.

The problems usually associated with the pattern of Lung dryness and Lung heat are generally superimposed on the previous pattern. Additional symptoms are listed above.

TREATMENT

▶ *Main Points*

TREATMENT PRINCIPLE: Nourish the yin, support the blood, and clear heat from the Lungs.

Local points	BL-1 (*jing ming*)	Brings qi to the eyes
	GB-1 (*tong zi liao*)	Brings qi to the eyes
	M-HN-5 (*tou guang ming*)	Brings qi to the eyes

Near points	TB-17 (yi feng)	Brings qi to the eyes
	GB-20 (feng chi)	Brings qi to the eyes
Distal points	ST-36 (zu san li)	Tonifies qi and blood
	BL-18 (gan shu)	Tonifies the Liver and Kidneys
	BL-23 (shen shu)	Tonifies the Liver and Kidneys

METHOD: The local points are needled superficially and gently with enough stimulation to feel the sensation in the front of the eye being treated. The near points are needled on the side of the affected eye, toward the eye. If the condition is bilateral, then both sides should be needled. The distal points are tonified, and the back associated points may be treated with needle and moxibustion.

▶ *Liver and Kidney Yin Deficiency*

In addition to the main points, add:

KI-3 (tai xi)	Tonifies the Kidney yin

METHOD: The tonifying method is used at the point.

▶ *Lung Dryness and Lung Heat*

In addition to the main points, add:

BL-13 (fei shu)	Moistens and cools the Lungs
LU-7 (lie que) and KI-6 (zhao hai)	This combination tonifies the yin of the entire body, especially that of the Lungs and Kidneys

METHOD: The tonifying method is used at all the points.

NOTE: In the case of Lung full heat, disperse LU-10 (yu ji).

RESULTS

The most significant progress can be seen in early-stage cataracts. If the cataract has only just started, there is a possibility of reversing it completely. Once the cataract has spread and the opacity has deepened, the chances of complete reversal are small. When the patient is old, progress will be slow. It should be possible to prevent the cataract from getting worse, but regular maintenance treatment will be needed.

Clinical study

I have not had the opportunity to treat a patient with cataracts. For this reason, I have included a summary of a clinical study reported in *Abstracts of Clinical Experience with Acupuncture* (pp. 303-304) on cataract patients. The points used included the following:

Local/near points	ST-1 *(cheng qi)*
	M-HN-8 *(qiu hou)*
	M-HN-9 *(tai yang)*
	M-HN-13 *(yi ming)*
	N-HN-3 *(jian ming)*
	N-HN-3(a) *(jian ming #1)*
	N-HN-3(d) *(jian ming #4)*
Distal points	LI-4 *(he gu)*
	ST-36 *(zu san li)*
	GB-37 *(guang ming)*
	BL-23 *(shen shu)*

In each treatment, two local/near points and one distal point, or one local/near point and two distal points were used. Treatment was given every day for 10 days, with a 5-day break. It is not recorded how many courses of treatment were given. The results are set forth in the following table.

Condition*	Marked Improvement	Some Improvement	No Change
Partial cataract (57)	26	30	1
Ripened cataract (16)	9	7	
Early cataract (17)	2	12	3
Cataract from external injury (6)		2	4

* The numbers in parentheses represent the total number of eyes for each condition.

COMMENT

The interesting thing about these results is that they show that acupuncture can make definite improvements in patients with cataracts. The cataract can be reversed to a certain extent, and thus acupuncture may be worthwhile if the patient cannot undergo cataract surgery. The results also show that there is a limit to the improvement that can be made.

What is not discussed in this study is the permanence of the beneficial effects of treatment, and whether maintenance acupuncture treatments are required. When treating a young person, it is possible to make permanent changes, but in an older person, maintenance treatment may be required on a regular basis.

Couching

The term 'couching' applies to a procedure that was carried out in the West and in China before the advent of eye surgery as we now know it. The technique was to insert a needle into the eye at the side and to mechanically sever the support of the opaque lens with the needle.

Couching is of benefit when the lens has become completely opaque, rendering the patient blind. When the lens is severed, the person can at least make out shapes, even if the shapes are extremely blurred. With the use of lenses, the individual's eyesight can be restored almost completely. Obviously, this method was not without its discomforts and dangers, and has now been superseded by laser surgery.

9.2 Near Sightedness (Myopia) in Children and Teenagers

Normal development of vision

When a baby is first born it has very little control over its vision. The eyes normally move together, and most of the time it seems that there is binocular vision. However, recent studies have shown that the focal length of the eyes is changing uncontrollably. As the baby gets older, he or she starts to develop control over both binocular vision and focus, but it is not until the child is about three-years old that the focus is reliable. In some children it may even be later than that. After this age, the eyesight should remain steady.

ONSET OF NEAR SIGHTEDNESS

Near sightedness is usually unnoticed until a child goes to school. It is generally picked up because the child appears to be backward, complains of not being able to see, or has headaches. This can happen at any age. It often happens when a child moves up a class or moves to a different school.

FURTHER DEVELOPMENT

The onset of near sightedness can occur at any age, but it likely occurs between age of 7 and 14 years. The longer it persists during the growing years, the more deeply ingrained it becomes. If the focus of the lens is too short during the years when the child is growing and the lens is hardening, then by the time the child's growth is complete, the eye will be 'set' into the wrong shape, and it will be difficult to change it back.

Western versus traditional approach

In conventional Western medicine, myopia is thought to be merely a structural problem: the unhappy combination of a lens that is too strong and an eyeball that is too large, resulting in imperfect focus. Consequently, any remedial action is taken on the mechanical level, that is, corrective lenses or mechanical alterations to the muscles or lens in the eye by laser treatment.

The traditional approach (in both the West and China) is that the eye is a part of a living organism and so can change. Like any other part of the body, if it is supplied with enough energy and exercised well, it will function perfectly. If some defect occurs, it is most likely a result of some impairment in the flow of energy and of overuse. Consequently, by returning the flow of energy to the eyes and by doing eye massages (see Chapter 6), near sightedness can often be cured.

TCM approach

ETIOLOGY

According to TCM theory, near sightedness has several causes. It may be there at birth—innate—or it can develop as a result of some problem in life, usually external stress or illness, or as a result of weak qi.

▶ *Innate*

Here the hereditary component can come from a familial tendency toward near sightedness, but what is most important is that some children really are born with eyes that are too long. Even from the earliest age, they are near sighted. If this is really significant (say more than 4 diopters[3]), there is little that can be done, and it is usually best for the child to wear spectacles. On the other hand, if this hereditary component is less than about 2 diopters, it may be worth trying to correct the condition by natural means.

▶ *Stress*

When a child has good vision that starts to deteriorate, this is nearly always a sign of some severe stress in the child's life. Common situations include:

- not getting on with the teacher
- afraid of the teacher
- moving to a new school or new class
- afraid of some impending event
- being bullied at school

There is a common emotion of fear and a common feeling that the child does not want to 'look' at the present or future situation.

▶ *Weak Qi*

In addition to stress, there is usually something that has weakened the child's qi. Common factors include:

- any illness that weakens the qi
- lingering pathogenic factor (from illness or immunization)
- exhaustion from overwork, television, and late nights
- straightforward Spleen qi deficiency

A NOTE ABOUT LINGERING PATHOGENIC FACTORS

The concept of a lingering pathogenic factor is explained more fully in *Acupuncture in the Treatment of Children* (3rd ed., p. 43). The idea is simple: a child becomes ill and never quite gets over it. There is always some slight trace of the original illness left in the body. Here are some characteristic signs and symptoms:

- slightly glazed look in the eyes
- lymph glands are swollen
- presence of thick phlegm, which is invisible for much of the time
- occasional abdominal aches for no apparent reason
- skin is abnormally rough in places
- occasionally, there is a powdery patch of skin on the cheek

The presence of the thick phlegm inhibits the flow of qi generally in the body. In this case, it may mean that the qi reaching the eyes is reduced.

TREATMENT

Treatment plays a role in countering two of the important causes of near sightedness:

Stress

Acupuncture has a great reputation for helping stressed-out adults, but in my opinion, this should not be its major role for children. Adults invariably will experience periods when the stress of life becomes intolerable, and acupuncture can be of great help in relieving stress and helping patients cope with difficulties in life. In children, acupuncture is also effective, but a much better principle is to arrange the lives of the children so that they only have realistic demands placed on them. When a child is under great stress, the aim of the treatment is to help the child and family identify the source of stress so that it can be resolved. An example from my own practice came from a child who developed near sightedness because he was being bullied at school. Treatment with acupuncture had short-term beneficial effects, but the cure came when he was given the Dr. Bach Flower Remedy 'Water Violet'. By giving this remedy frequently, he became less aloof and withdrawn, and so the school bully no longer felt the need to attack him.

Weak qi

As mentioned above, weak qi can arise because of straightforward Spleen qi deficiency or a lingering pathogenic factor.

▶ *Main Points*

Undoubtedly, the best way to bring qi to the eyes is for the child to do the self-massage techniques described in Section 6.2. There are two additional ways of bringing qi to the eyes: acupuncture and the electric plum blossom method (also described in Section 6.2).

The points to use are:

Local points	BL-2 (*zan shu*)
	M-HN-6 (*yu yao*)
	TB-23 (*si zhu kong*)
	ST-2 (*si bai*)
Near point	GB-2 (*ting hui*)
Distal points	LI-4 (*he gu*)
	PC-6 (*nei guan*) (optional)

Ideally, these points are treated every day for 10 days, with a rest of 5 days. In practice, they should be treated minimally three times a week. Less frequent treatments are not worth doing and just lead to frustration and expense on the part of the parents.

▶ *Spleen Qi Deficiency*

In addition to the main points, add:

ST-36 *(zu san li)*	Tonifies the Stomach and Spleen qi
SP-6 *(san yin jiao)*	Tonifies the Spleen and Kidneys

METHOD: The tonifying method is used at these points.

▶ *Lingering Pathogenic Factor*

Once the Spleen weakness has been overcome, there may still be a lingering pathogenic factor. A typical treatment for this would include the following main points, as needed:

M-HN-30 *(bai lao)*	Clears the lingering pathogenic factor
BL-18 *(gan shu)*	Softens thick phlegm associated with a lingering pathogenic factor
BL-20 *(pi shu)*	Softens thick phlegm associated with a lingering pathogenic factor

METHOD: The even or moving technique is used at these points.

WHEN TO USE THE ELECTRIC PLUM BLOSSOM METHOD

Some children will take well to eye massage. Even quite young children take pride in doing them and will not let anything get in the way. Others are monstrously lazy and need cajoling and persuading to do anything that will help their eyesight. For these children, regular treatment and the status gained by regular visits to a practitioner can be helpful in giving them the impetus to do at least *some* exercises.

SELF-CHECKING

When the children do the exercises, or following a treatment, there is usually an immediate improvement in the eyesight. It is helpful for the child and the parents (and possibly the practitioner) to see this actually happening, and so it is a good idea to set up a simple eye test just before doing the treatment (or the exercise) and then again immediately after the treatment. The detectable change will give everyone encouragement.

MAINTAINING QI IN THE EYES AFTER TREATMENTS

The best way (in fact, the only way) to maintain the flow of qi to the eyes is to use them. The child should be encouraged to look carefully at pictures and at scenes, and to generally look carefully at their surroundings. The very act of looking brings qi to the eyes.

AUTHOR'S EXPERIENCE

I have treated many cases of near sightedness, mostly with success.

Advice to parents

- Always make sure the child has good light when reading or doing close work. Using the eyes often in poor light causes eye strain.
- Do not let the child watch television or do computer games. Both of these activities are injurious to weak eyes, not only from the flickering, blurred images, but from the level of tension that results.
- Make sure the child sits in a good position when doing close work. Reading or writing in a cramped position inhibits the flow of qi to the eyes and is likely to lead to eye strain.
- Make sure the child spends some time each day without spectacles (if the child wears spectacles constantly). Also, gradually reduce the strength of the spectacles rather than gradually increasing it.

Conclusion

The methods described here work especially well in children. Even adults, if they are determined enough, can throw away their spectacles or contacts. It is sad that spectacles are always prescribed without even a thought for developing good eyesight. It is possible that 9 out of 10 people who now wear glasses would not need them if treatment had been given at the right time and with the appropriate method.

Endnotes

1. This is an analogy that is often used, and it is a fair analogy for describing the process at the molecular level, that is, changes in the shape and perhaps size of the proteins. Moreover, the most common pattern seen in cataract patients is that of heat, so one can literally think of the lens of the eye being 'cooked' in much the same way as an egg.

2. If the patient is taking medication for high blood pressure, the known side effects of the medication should be checked for there are some medications that lead to cataract.

3. A diopter is a unit used in optics to measure the strength of a lens. In ophthalmology, it has a slightly different meaning, and it measures the degree of imperfection of the lens of the eye. So, for example, +1 diopter would be slightly near sighted, and +2 is a bit more near sighted. To correct near sightedness of +2 diopters, a concave lens would be prescribed of -2 diopters. A lens of 1 diopter has a focal length of 1 meter (approximately 39 inches), and a lens of 2 diopters has a focal length of 50 centimeters (approximately 19 inches).

Chapter 10

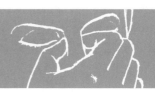

Problems of the Front of the Eye

Section 10.1 provides an overview of conjunctivitis. The three categories of conjunctivitis—acute conjunctivitis, chronic conjunctivitis, and conjunctivitis as a result of hay fever—are discussed separately in Sections 10.2 to 10.4. Three related corneal conditions—corneal ulcers, opacity, and erosion—are discussed in Section 10.5. Two less commonly seen problems of the front of the eye—pinguecula and blepharitis—are discussed in Sections 10.6 and 10.7.

10.1   Conjunctivitis: An Introduction

Conjunctivitis is an inflammation of the conjunctiva of the eye (Fig. 10.1). The general symptoms of conjunctivitis include:

- pinkish, reddish, or sometimes blood-shot eye, which is said to be the result of inflammation of the blood vessels of the conjunctiva
- gritty, sore eye
- possibly discharge of pus
- eyelids may be 'gummed' together after sleep
- oversensitivity to light

The severity of the problem varies from a single mildly itching eye to both eyes being red and painful. In addition, the problem can range from an occasional acute attack to a chronic condition that has been around for months or years.

Acute conjunctivitis is a sudden inflammation of the conjunctiva of the eye. Chronic conjunctivitis is a chronic inflammation of the conjunctiva with exacerbation of the symptoms and periods of remission that last over months or years. The causes are said to be the same as for acute conjunctivitis. Conjunctivitis is also a symptom of hay fever, but the nature of the allergy in hay fever and the regularity of its timing set it apart from straightforward conjunctivitis.

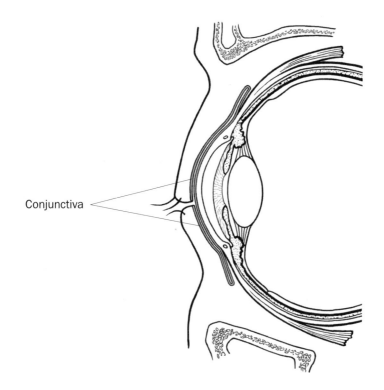

Conjunctiva

Fig. 10.1 The conjunctiva

Acupuncture can be very helpful in the treatment of each condition. In an acute attack, the itching and discomfort can often be reduced in just one treatment. In chronic conditions where the problem is more long-standing, the condition can often be cured over the course of some 20 treatments.

10.2 Acute Conjunctivitis

Etiology

Acute conjunctivitis is attributed to a viral or bacterial infection or as a result of an 'allergic reaction'. The viral form is known as 'pinkeye' while the red, irritated eye is usually associated with a bacterial infection. Conjunctivitis caused by these two infectious agents is believed to be contagious, and good hygiene—for example, keeping the hands away from the eyes, washing the hands, washing sheets and pillowcases in hot water, and not sharing eye-related paraphernalia—is believed to be essential for controlling the spread of the disease. Conjunctivitis that results from an allergic reaction is believed not to be contagious. Common allergens include pollen, animal hair or dander, dust, chemicals, and certain medications.

TCM approach

ETIOLOGY AND PATHOLOGY

There are two common patterns of acute conjunctivitis: wind-heat and uprising heat and dampness. The former is a straightforward invasion of wind-heat attacking the eyes, which can be caused by exposure to extremes of temperature, either hot or cold, especially if this is combined with exposure to wind. This combination is found among those who spend a large amount of time on bicycles. The eye problem can also be caused by an attack of influenza. The invading wind disrupts the flow of qi and fluids. Signs and symptoms of this pattern include:

- red, sore, itchy eyes
- possibly watering eyes
- sudden onset
- signs of an attack of wind-heat
- possible fever
- possible thirst
- floating and rapid pulse
- tongue has thin coating and red tip

If wind is the predominant component in these patients, there will be an increase in watery secretions. If heat is the predominant component, redness and pain will be more pronounced.

In the pattern of uprising heat and dampness, interior heat and dampness rise up to the eye, causing it to become red and painful, and to discharge sticky, yellow matter.[1] The common causes of this pattern include:

- a diet rich in spicy, greasy foods
- a diet of poor-quality food, containing preservatives and colorings
- strong feelings of anger and aggression that lead to the restraint of Liver qi
- latent heat in the springtime

Signs and symptoms of this pattern include:

- eyes are red and painful
- yellow, sticky discharge from the eyes
- possible yellow nasal discharge
- possible indigestion
- greasy and dirty looking tongue coating
- tongue body is red, especially at the sides
- slippery and rapid pulse

Note that this pattern is commonly seen in bacterial conjunctivitis. In addition, it often combines with the wind-heat pattern.

TREATMENT

▶ *Main Points*

The following prescription is helpful in all acute attacks:

GB-20 *(feng chi)*	Clears wind and heat and brightens the eyes
LI-4 *(he gu)*	Clears wind and brings qi to the eyes (via the channel)
GB-37 *(guang ming)*	Benefits the eyes and clears heat

Other useful points include:

GV-23 *(shang xing)*	Brings qi to the eyes
TB-3 *(zhong zhu)*	Very good for mild attacks of conjunctivitis; does not interfere too much with the patient's qi circulation
M-HN-10 *(er jian)*	Clears pain and redness in the eyes

METHOD: Use a reducing method at all the points.

▶ *Wind-Heat*

TREATMENT PRINCIPLE: Clear the wind-heat and cool and nourish the eyes.

LU-7 (*lie que*)	Clears wind-heat
TB-5 (*wai guan*)	Clears wind-heat
M-HN-9 (*tai yang*)	Clears wind-heat affecting the head

If there is very high fever, add:

LI-1 (*shang yang*)	Clears extreme heat

If the eyes are very red, add:

PC-7 (*da ling*)	'Experience' point for red eyes

If the fever, inflammation, and pain are only mild, then just the following point may be enough:

TB-3 (*zhong zhu*)	Clears red eyes

PROGNOSIS: Two or three treatments should be enough. The patient may break out into a sweat as the pathogenic factor is expelled.

▶ *Uprising Heat and Dampness*

TREATMENT PRINCIPLE: Clear the heat and dampness from the eyes.

As noted above, the points GB-20 (*feng chi*), LI-4 (*he gu*), and GB-37 (*guang ming*) should be used. If there is obvious dampness and discharge in the eye, add:

GB-34 (*yang ling quan*)	Clears phlegm-dampness from the Liver and Gallbladder

PROGNOSIS: The number of treatments that will be required depends on the cause, but one to three treatments should be enough to clear the eyes. However, treatment should continue long enough to resolve any underlying problem, including the patient's diet. For example, if there are signs of pus, the patient should avoid eating eggs.

Western medical and acupuncture treatment

The conventional Western medical treatment depends on the cause. If the inflammation is due to a viral infection, the patient is told to simply wait until the condition runs its course—usually one to two weeks. If the inflammation is due to a bacterial invasion, antibiotic eye drops are usually given. The bacteria are considered to be very contagious, so the patient is normally kept isolated from other people, for example, children should be kept at home. If the inflammation is believed to be the result of an allergic reaction, a short course of topical corticosteroids and antibiotics is usually prescribed.[2]

I have treated many cases of acute conjunctivitis in children with remarkable success. I have not had the opportunity to treat the condition in adults but would imagine that the results would be comparable.

Welder's eye

There is another pattern of acute conjunctivitis that is rarely seen by acupuncturists and is known colloquially as 'welder's eye'. This form of conjunctivitis is a result of the eye being exposed to intense ultraviolet radiation, such as would be experienced by an arc welder who was not using an eye shield. Symptoms include:

- intense pain in the eye, which persists for about three days and then usually subsides on its own
- extreme bloodshot eye

The treatment of this condition would be the same as for the wind-heat pattern given above.

Welder's eye is mentioned in many of the Chinese acupuncture texts (under the heading 'electric ophthyalmia'). Acupuncture is apparently very effective in reducing the pain and inflammation of this condition. In *Abstracts of Clinical Experience with Acupuncture* (p. 297), the following results are given for a single acupuncture treatment in 46 cases of welder's eye: 37 were pain free after the treatment, and 9 had no relief. Even if the research methodology does not stand up to the criteria of modern science, the results claimed are nevertheless very striking.

10.3   Chronic Conjunctivitis

Chronic conjunctivitis is a chronic inflammation of the conjunctiva with exacerbation of the symptoms and periods of remission that last over months or years. Often the inflammation and pain are not as severe as in acute conjunctivitis, but the continuing discomfort can be depressing.

Etiology

The chronic condition is often a result of a persistence of the acute condition. It is also thought that the condition is a result of chronic exposure to an irritant or is a secondary reaction to, say, blepharitis (see Section 10.7) and entropion (see Section 12.5). The irritant may be a consequence of overtreatment with medications, resulting in drug-induced sensitivity.

TCM approach

ETIOLOGY AND PATHOLOGY

There are two commonly seen patterns:

- Liver and Gallbladder heat
- Liver and Kidney weakness

The most common cause of Liver and Gallbladder heat is constrained emotions, particularly anger. Additional contributing factors include a diet that is rich in greasy, hot, or spicy foods, alcohol, and smoking. The heat and dampness enter the Liver and Gallbladder channels and rise up to the eyes. Signs and symptoms of this pattern include:

- eyes alternate between normal and being red, swollen, and painful
- red face
- possibly has strong smelling, highly colored, scanty urine, especially when the eyes are inflamed
- often worse when the patient is upset or angry
- red tongue
- wiry pulse

It is said that the symptoms of the weak pattern of chronic conjunctivitis appear because the qi in the eyes is weak, which opens the way for wind to enter the eyes and cause redness and itching. The weakness of qi in the eyes is usually a result of weakness in the Liver and Kidney organs themselves. This can happen in old age. It is also seen in patients who repress their anger, but instead of becoming more and more aggressive, they become more and more introverted. In some patients, especially the young, the pattern arises because the channels are blocked, for example, by a lingering pathogenic factor so that little qi reaches the eyes. Signs and symptoms of this pattern include:

- eyes are often causing problems
- eyes look dull and maybe watery
- patient is listless and without energy.
- pulse is weak or thready, or maybe weak and soft

In both of these chronic patterns, the eyes and the area around the eyes have a dull appearance. It seems as though the eyes are sitting in a dull, gray pool.

TREATMENT

▶ *Main Points*

Points to bring qi to the eyes include:

BL-1 *(jing ming)*
GB-20 *(feng chi)*
LI-4 *(he gu)*

METHOD: The even method is used a all these points.

▶ *Liver and Gallbladder Heat*

TREATMENT PRINCIPLE: Clear damp-heat from the Liver and Gallbladder. In addition to the main points, add:

M-HN-9 *(tai yang)*	Clears Heat affecting the head
LR-2 *(xing jian)*	Clears Liver heat and brightens the eyes
LR-3 *(tai chong)*	Clears Liver heat and brightens the eyes
GB-37 *(guang ming)*	Brightens the eyes

METHOD: The even method is used at the main points and a strong dispersing method at the other points.

ADVICE: The patient should be encouraged to avoid eating greasy, spicy foods and using too much alcohol, and to take plenty of exercise, preferably in the fresh air.

► *Liver and Kidney Weakness*

TREATMENT PRINCIPLE: Tonify the Liver and Kidneys and firm the original (*yuan*) QI.

In addition to the main points, use those below since they are good for organ and channel weakness:

ST-36 (*zu san li*)	Tonifies the original qi
LR-3 (*tai chong*)	Tonifies the Liver and Kidneys and brightens the eyes
BL-18 (*gan shu*)	Tonifies the Liver and Kidney
BL-20 (*pi shu*)	Tonifies the Spleen and Liver
BL-23 (*shen shu*)	Tonifies the Liver and Kidneys

METHOD: The tonifying method is used at all the points. Moxibustion can be used at the back associated points.

PROGNOSIS: This varies depending on the level of exhaustion of the patient. If the exhaustion is of recent origin, 20 treatments may be enough. In some cases, treatment may need to continue longer.

Western medical and acupuncture treatment

There is not much that Western medicine has to offer for the treatment of chronic conjunctivitis. Obviously, irritating factors are to be eliminated, including perhaps medications that the patient is taking. Some medical texts suggest the prophylactic stimulation of the meibomium glands under carefully controlled conditions. In addition, topical corticosteroids and antibiotic therapy is often prescribed.

I have treated a handful of cases with chronic conjunctivitis as the main presenting symptoms, and many more where it was a secondary symptom. When it is the main symptom, it responds slowly but surely. In addition, there were no unforeseen setbacks. When it was a secondary symptom, some improvement was noted, but the patient did not usually stay until that particular symptom had healed. Note that rest is essential, as is a good diet containing fresh organic foods.

10.4   Hay Fever[3]

Hay fever is a seasonal irritation of the mucous membranes of the eyes, nose, and occasionally the upper respiratory tract. In the long distant past, hay fever was a real fever that people got when they were making hay or were near others who were making hay. Over the years its meaning has changed, so that now it has come to mean allergic rhinitis. In some patients the problems arise at specific times of year, while in others it arises on exposure to specific allergens such as hay dust or particular pollens, for example, grass pollens or the pollen from rape flowers. Typical symptoms include:

- nasal congestion and irritation, with discharge
- sneezing
- red, watery eyes

Often, there is

- difficulty concentrating
- thick mucous discharge
- headache
- photophobia
- irritable cough

The onset is seasonal and is usually identified with pollen of various sorts, with some people being more upset by grass pollens (summer type) and some more by pollens from flowers and trees (spring type). For some people the sheer joy of seeing an old-fashioned meadow full of flowers is replaced by the sheer misery of hay fever. And for some, the effect is so violent that they have to stay indoors for a few weeks. Others have adopted drastic solutions like wearing a sort of space suit when they are outside with a Perspex pollen-free dome around their head!

Sources

I have not found any clear descriptions of hay fever beyond the standard ones describing conjunctivitis. Therefore, what follows is based on clinical experience. Inevitably, it is one-sided, being based on the hay fever patients who have visited the clinic.

TCM approach

The emphasis in TCM is on internal factors. Although hay fever appears at a certain time of year, it is related more to the time than to the pollen. In fact, the time of onset—both the time of the year and the age in years when hay fever started—provides a pointer to the etiology and pathology.

TIME OF YEAR

The time of year, late spring to early summer, when many patients suffer from hay fever is marked by a change of season from cold to hot. The hottest days have not yet been reached, and the average temperature is still increasing. If the Liver's function of ensuring the free flow of qi is at all faulty, then the body will not adapt quickly enough. As a result, the warmth that has been stored in winter will remain through the spring and manifest as heat, a phenomenon known as 'latent heat.'

TIME OF LIFE

Hay fever is rare before the age of five, and this provides a further clue. This is the age when the emotions start to become controllable. It is also the age when stagnation of Liver qi first appears. Before this age, there is little in the way of restraint of emotions, and so the incidence of hay fever is very low.

ETIOLOGY AND PATHOLOGY

The particles of pollen or other allergen are the external trigger for an attack. The internal factor is stagnation of qi in the eyes and nose, which can be a result of any of the following patterns:

- Liver yang rising
- Liver and Gallbladder damp-heat
- lingering pathogenic factor
- Lung and Spleen qi deficiency
- Lung and Kidney deficiency

Thus, the local stagnation of qi may be due to fire rising up, as in Liver yang rising, local stagnation, as in a lingering pathogenic factor, or insufficient qi overall, as in the remaining patterns.

There is yet another underlying cause not mentioned in either the Western or Chinese texts, and that is the effects of mercury leaching from dental fillings.

As the mercury slowly drains upward, it can severely affect the eye, exacerbating each of the listed patterns by causing local stagnation and irritation (see Appendix 3).

▶ *Liver Yang Rising*

The restraint of the 'seven emotions' for any length of time impairs the Liver's function of ensuring the free flow of qi, resulting in qi stagnation.[4] Over a period of time, the stagnation transforms to heat and leads to Liver yang rising, which rises up to the eyes and nose and causes local heat and stagnation. Signs and symptoms include:

- red and/or watering eyes and other symptoms of hay fever
- frequently flies into a rage
- face color may be red or white but becomes purple when enraged
- purple tongue
- wiry pulse

▶ *Liver and Gallbladder Damp-Heat*

Damp-heat may accumulate due to a variety of causes, such as the overconsumption of spicy foods, excess sugary foods, or meat and alcohol, or an intolerance to gluten. Sometimes it is a result of a combination of restrained emotions and a damp climate, as we experience in England. Once the damp-heat has accumulated, it can rise up to the eyes and nose and cause the irritation characteristic of hay fever. Signs and symptoms include:

- red and/or watering eyes and other symptoms of hay fever
- yellow-green nasal discharge
- irritability
- dull gray face, somewhat puffy, or dusky red face
- tongue coating is yellow and slimy, tongue body tends to be red
- slippery and rapid pulse

▶ *Lingering Pathogenic Factor*

A lingering pathogenic factor is the remains of an illness that the patient had earlier. Often this pattern is caused by the remains of an old Lung infection. The infection is never completely thrown out, leaving behind the traces of illness that affect the Lung system. This manifests as irritation of the mucous membranes, which is characteristic of a subacute inflammation. Typical of this pattern is the presence of very thick phlegm; sometimes it is so thick that it is not apparent at first. Signs and symptoms include:

- red and/or watering eyes and other symptoms of hay fever
- often a gentle demeanor
- possible dry cough from time to time
- slightly glazed look in the eyes
- greasy skin
- gray face or sometimes red face
- pulse may be slippery or weaker[5]

▶ *Lung and Spleen Qi Deficiency*

In the past this pattern commonly arose from overwork or from a long illness. Now it often arises early in childhood as a result of a variety of causes, including a difficult birth, irregular feeding during childhood, or overimmunization. Once the pattern has taken hold it may remain with the patient for life. If the qi is weak, then once stagnation has arisen in the Lung system, for example, from a cold in the nose, then there is not enough qi for the body to recover completely. Signs and symptoms include:

- red and/or watering eyes and other symptoms of hay fever
- droopy, cannot stand up straight
- probably poor appetite
- white face
- weak pulse
- pale tongue body

▶ *Lung and Kidney Deficiency*

The term 'deficiency' rather than 'yin deficiency' is given for this pattern because the modern presentation is a combination of yin and yang deficiency. The pattern often starts early in life, mainly as Lung and Spleen qi deficiency, at which point a combination of overwork and insufficient sleep can lead to Kidney weakness. If there is the slightest amount of heat in the system, this may rise up to the eyes and nose, presenting with local inflammation and irritation. If the patient does a lot of physical work, there may be the classic signs of yin deficiency with malar flush and night sweats. However, it is more common to find that the patient has become overtired from mental work, in which case these characteristic signs may be absent. Signs and symptoms include:

- red and/or watering eyes and other symptoms of hay fever
- thin body
- dark pools around the eyes
- weak back
- stays up late and is overstimulated and overworked
- very pale, possibly with red cheeks
- rapid pulse

TREATMENT

▶ *Main Points*

The following prescription is good for all types of hay fever. These points are particularly effective during an acute attack when they should be strongly dispersed.

LU-7 *(lie que)*	Tonifies the Lungs, clears phlegm, and opens the nose
LI-4 *(he gu)*	Benefits the nose, face, and face
LI-20 *(ying xiang)*	Local point for the nose, tonifies the Lungs, and brings qi to the eyes

Note: There are two other commonly used points:

GB-39 *(xuan zhong)*	Benefits the nose and eyes and brings down Liver yang
LR-3 *(tai chong)*	Regulates the Liver

These points are helpful during the season when the main thrust of treatment is to relieve the symptoms. When treating in advance of the season, more emphasis should be given to treating the underlying pattern.

▶ *Liver Yang Rising*

TREATMENT PRINCIPLE: Clear heat in the eyes and subdue Liver yang.
In addition to the main points, add:

LR-2 *(xing jian)*	Brings down Liver yang
LR-3 *(tai chong)*	Brings down Liver yang
LI-4 *(he gu)*	Calms Liver yang, brings qi to the eyes, and opens the nose

METHOD: The strong dispersion technique is used at the points.

RESULTS: These points can have a very calming effect on the patient. In some cases the ensuing calm allows the patients to examine their lives and to take the necessary steps to avoid becoming as stressed again. In other cases, regular maintenance treatments are beneficial.

▶ *Lingering Pathogenic Factor*

TREATMENT PRINCIPLE: Clear the eyes and eliminate the lingering pathogenic factor.

In addition to the main points, add:

M-HN-30 *(bai lao)*	Loosens thick phlegm
BL-18 *(gan shu)*	Loosens thick phlegm and eases the free flow of Liver qi
BL-20 *(pi shu)*	Loosens and resolves phlegm
ST-40 *(feng long)*	Resolves phlegm

METHOD: The even technique is used at all the points.

RESULTS: If these points are used outside the hay fever season, there is the possibility of eliminating the lingering pathogenic factor, but it will take time. An early sign that the treatments are working is that the dry nose will become wetter, with discharge of thick phlegm.

▶ *Liver and Gallbladder Damp-Heat*

TREATMENT PRINCIPLE: Clear the eyes and eliminate Liver and Gallbladder damp-heat.

In addition to the main points, add:

LR-13 *(zhang men)*	Resolves Liver and Gallbladder damp-heat
CV-12 *(zhong wan)*	Moves the qi and benefits the Spleen to resolve dampness
GB-34 *(yang ling quan)*	Resolves Liver and Gallbladder damp-heat
GB-39 *(xuan zhong)*	Benefits the eyes and nose and brings down Liver yang

METHOD: The even or dispersing method is used at all the points.

RESULTS: The symptoms can easily be relieved during the season if treatment is given once a week. Although this is basically a condition of excess, it can be surprisingly difficult to eliminate the pattern altogether and provide a complete cure.

▶ *Lung and Spleen Qi Deficiency*

TREATMENT PRINCIPLE: Bring qi to the eyes and tonify the Lung and Spleen. In addition to the main points, add:

LU-7 (*lie que*)	Tonifies the Lungs and opens the nose
ST-36 (*zu san li*)	Tonifies the Spleen
SP-6 (*san yin jiao*)	Tonifies the Spleen

METHOD: The tonifying method is used at all the points

RESULTS: The time it takes to cure this condition depends on the patient's level of deficiency. If they are very deficient and the problem has been there a long time, it will take many treatments. If the deficiency is not so significant and the organs are only mildly affected, the problem may be cured in one or two seasons. In the meantime, the symptoms of hay fever can be controlled during the season if treatment is given once a week.

▶ *Lung and Kidney Deficiency*

TREATMENT PRINCIPLE: Bring qi to the eyes and tonify the Lungs and Kidneys. In addition to the main points, add:

LU-7 (*lie que*)	Tonifies the Lungs and opens the nose
BL-23 (*shen shu*)	Strengthens the Kidneys
KI-3 (*tai xi*)	Tonifies the Kidneys as well as the Kidney yin

METHOD: The tonifying method is used at all the points.

RESULTS: By its very nature, this pattern is deep and of long duration. Therefore, it is likely to require many treatments and a long time to cure. However, the symptoms of red eyes during the hay fever season can be controlled by acupuncture.

Western medical and acupuncture treatment

In Western medicine, hay fever is seen as an allergic histamine response to foreign bodies that attack the conjunctiva and the lining of the nasal cavity. The emphasis is on the external attacking agent, identifying the pollen as an outside invading force. The treatment is of two types: desensitization treatments and antihistamine-based treatments. They both have some drawbacks. The desensitizing treatment is quite variable in its results and can occasionally lead to anaphylactic shock. The antihistamine-based treatment may make the patient feel drowsy.

Acupuncture usually provides excellent relief of symptoms during an attack, and if treatment is given before the pollen-producing season, there is even better success. The best time to treat these patients is four to six weeks before the hay fever season, which is in the middle of spring and is the ideal time to treat all Liver-related diseases. Two or three treatments at this time can make a huge difference in the severity of the symptoms later on.

That being said, curing the underlying pattern so that the symptoms never return is not so easy. Some patients respond very well, and treating these individuals over two or three seasons is enough to cure the problem once and for all. In other patients, there are difficulties. These arise because they may need to make significant internal changes, and the magnitude of these changes may seem to them to be out of proportion to the severity of the symptoms. For example, if the underlying cause is a difficult relationship with the patient's spouse, the internal and external changes needed may be very large. Subconsciously, the person feels that it is better to muddle along and suffer some minor symptoms rather than go through the upheavals that may arise when deep changes are made to the structure of the marriage.

10.5   Corneal Ulcer, Opacity, and Erosion

Corneal ulcer is the name given to localized opacity of the cornea (Fig. 10.2), while corneal opacity is the name given to generalized opacity and clouding of the cornea.[6] Corneal erosion is the name given when the cornea becomes damaged.

The general symptoms of corneal ulcer and opacity include:

• localized opacity
• nearby redness and excess blood vessels

- photophobia
- watering eyes
- pain similar to that felt with a foreign body
- irritable iritis (because toxins reach the iris)

The symptoms of corneal erosion are similar, but the pain is more severe.

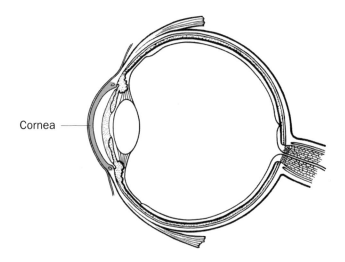

Cornea

Fig. 10.2 The cornea

It may be thought that corneal ulcer and opacity cannot be treated by acupuncture, that it is like using a needle to clear a cloudy windscreen. In fact, the situation is different, and acupuncture can be very effective. As explained in the following paragraphs, there is a 'body condition' underlying the various corneal disorders, and by changing the body condition and bringing qi to the eyes, the eyes will heal themselves.

Once again, several Western medical categories of disease are grouped together for the purpose of discussion according to Chinese medicine. And once again this is partly due to the inadequacies of traditional ophthalmology and partly due to the completely different way conditions are classified in Western and Chinese medicine. We will therefore see that two patients who have the same diagnosis in Western medicine might have different diagnoses in Chinese medicine, and vice versa. When using Chinese medicine, it is essential to use Chinese medical diagnoses.

Etiology

The cornea is hard and surprisingly robust since it is made of closely packed sheets of cells. It is, however, vulnerable to a disturbance in its fluid balance, and this is how most of the problems with the cornea arise. As a result of an imbalance, the closely packed layers become slightly separated by fluid layers. The result is that the normally clear cornea becomes slightly milky and opaque. In this, there are certain similarities with eczema, a fact that explains why there is a Lung pattern for this condition.

Western medical classification of corneal ulcer

Cause	Description
Bacterial infection	Often the bacteria are 'opportunistic' in that they invade the cornea after it has been injured. However, sometimes they just come for no known reason.
Marginal ulcers	This type is seen most frequently in middle-aged women. It is painful but benign.
Herpes simplex infection	The virus invades the epithelium, which then ruptures, leading to dendritic ulcers.
Herpes zoster infection	This virus invades the cornea, giving rise to neuralgic pain.
Other viral infections	Infection by other viruses, such as adenovirus or the paramyxovirus responsible for measles, can also result in corneal ulcer.
Fungal infections	'Indolent' ulcers are assumed to be fungal in origin until proven otherwise.

From the point of view of Western medicine, the disturbance that causes this opacity is nearly always an infection from the outside, either bacterial, viral, or fungal, and the usual array of antibiotics, antivirals, and antifungals are used to treat the conditions with varying degrees of success.

TCM approach

Once again, Chinese medicine has a wider perspective. The role of exogenous pathogenic factors is recognized, but so also is the role played by the body's strength and its ability or inability to resist disease. This is clearly seen in the following differentiation of patterns:

- Liver and Kidney weakness (or Liver and Kidney yin deficiency)
- Liver and Gallbladder heat
- Wind-heat
- Lung yin deficiency

In this list, only the wind-heat pattern reflects an attack by an external pathogenic factor. Again, there is yet another underlying cause not mentioned in either the Western or Chinese texts and that is the effects of mercury leaking from dental fillings. As the mercury slowly drains upward, it can severely affect the eye, predisposing the cornea to ulcer and erosion (see Appendix 3).

ETIOLOGY AND PATHOLOGY

▶ *Liver and Kidney Weakness*

I prefer the expression 'Liver and Kidney weakness' to 'Liver and Kidney yin deficiency', although both terms are correct. The corneal opacity arises because of weak heat—hence the use of yin deficiency—but frequently the patients do not have many of the characteristic signs that one would expect of yin deficiency, such as malar flush, night sweats, and so on. What is more common is that the patients will appear to be worn out. The overall weakness of both Kidney yin and yang will be evident in their appearance. Likewise, the Liver weakness will show in typical signs such as creakiness of the joints, irritability, and lack of flexibility. Signs and symptoms include:

- sclera has a 'muddy' look
- patient is tired
- weak knees
- sore or weak back
- pasty complexion
- tongue may be pale, possibly with red at the edges
- soggy and weak pulse

▶ *Liver and Gallbladder Heat*

This is known in some books as 'Liver channel obstructed heat,' and this is a good description of the pattern in a sizeable portion of the patients. The heat may indeed arise from true Liver heat, and there may be the tell-tale signs of, say, hypochondriac pain. However, the pattern is more likely seen in a fairly strong patient without really strong Liver signs. There may be signs of stagnation, with local development of heat, but rarely does one see the explosive anger, red face, and red tongue associated with Liver heat. Signs and symptoms include:

- bloodshot eyes
- possibly a red face, but more often in the West, the face is pale
- male patients may have blue color along the jawline
- tense and irritable
- tendency to high blood pressure
- wiry pulse
- purple tongue

▶ *Wind-Heat*

This is more straightforward and corresponds to a sudden infection that results in a severe case of acute conjunctivitis, which progresses, leading to changes in the cornea. At the time of the invasion of wind-heat, there is significant fever. Signs and symptoms include those of acute conjunctivitis, including:

- very red, very sore, itchy eyes
- possibly watery eyes
- sudden onset
- signs of an attack of wind-heat
- possible fever
- possible thirst
- pulse is floating and rapid
- tongue has thin coating and red tip

▶ *Lung Yin Deficiency*

As mentioned in the introduction to this section, the cornea, as an extension of the sclera, pertains to the Lungs. In some sense, the cornea may be thought of as analogous to the skin. Consequently, a disease of the cornea may be related to a Lung imbalance. In China, Lung yin deficiency occurs as a result of the after effects of serious Lung diseases, including progressive tuberculosis. In the West, Lung yin deficiency is likely to be seen as a result of conditions like asthma or persistent overwork. Signs and symptoms include:

- white face with malar flush
- night sweats
- thin build
- history of Lung problems
- possible history of excessive use of steroids for treating asthma
- overstimulated
- pulse is fine and rapid
- tongue is thin, red at tip or red all over, and maybe peeled

TREATMENT

The following prescriptions— without accompanying treatment principle or needle technique—are set forth in *Practical Acupuncture* (1982):

▶ *Corneal Ulcer and Corneal Opacity*

Prescription 1	Prescription 2
BL-1 *(jing ming)*	BL-2 *(zan zhu)*
GB-14 *(yang bai)*	ST-2 *(si bai)*
M-HN-9 *(tai yang)*	M-HN-6 *(yu yao)*
M-HN-10 *(er jian)*	CV-17 *(ju que)*
LI-4 *(he gu)*	GV-23 *(shen shu)*
BL-18 *(gan shu)*	

▶ *Corneal Erosion*

The following prescriptions are given according to the pattern. For Liver and Kidney weakness, use:

BL-1 *(jing ming)*	Brings qi to the eyes
BL-2 *(zan zhu)*	Brings qi to the eyes
M-HN-9 *(tai yang)*	Brings qi to the eyes
BL-18 *(gan shu)*	Strengthens the Liver and Kidneys
LR-1 *(da dun)*	Benefits the Liver and clears heat from the eyes
BL-23 *(shen shu)*	Strengthens the Liver and Kidneys

For Liver and Gallbladder heat, use:

BL-1 (jing ming)	Clears heat from the eyes
M-HN-9 (tai yang)	Clears heat from the eyes
SP-1 (yin bai)*	Clears Liver and Gallbladder damp-heat and benefits the eyes
BL-18 (gan shu)	Clears Liver and Gallbladder damp-heat and benefits the eyes
LR-13 (zhang men)	Clears Liver and Gallbladder damp-heat and benefits the eyes

* Note that this point is bled.

For wind-heat, use:

BL-1 (jing ming)	Clears heat from the eyes
M-HN-9 (tai yang)	Clears heat from the eyes and head
GB-20 (feng chi)	Expels wind and brightens the eyes

For Lung yin deficiency, use:

BL-13 (fei shu)	Tonifies the Lung yin
LU-1 (zhong fu)	Clears heat from the Lungs
LU-9 (tai yuan)	Tonifies the Lungs
LU-6 (kong zui)	Regulates the Lungs

CLINICAL STUDY

The following results are reported in *Abstracts of Clinical Experience with Acupuncture* (p. 289). Out of a total of 38 eyes treated, 34 were much improved, 3 were slightly improved, and 1 had no change. The treatment given was quite extensive, involving 1 to 3 courses of 10 treatments each.

Western medical and acupuncture treatment

Bacterial ulcers are treated with antibiotic eye drops, which are usually successful. At the present time, when most bacteria are not yet resistant to antibiotics, this is the appropriate initial treatment. It would be irresponsible to deny anyone this simple treatment unless the individual has a history of adverse reactions to antibiotics. The role of acupuncture is then to support the body so that the problem does not return. In terms of Western medicine, this would mean strengthening the immune system. In terms of Chinese medicine, this means bringing qi to the eyes and correcting the underlying imbalance.

Viral ulcers are treated with antivirals, but with only limited success. Here the role of acupuncture is much greater, for by bringing qi to the eyes and regulating the body condition, there is a good chance that the immune system will be sufficiently invigorated to expel the virus completely.

Acupuncture should certainly be considered if the opacity does not respond to Western medical treatment. Moreover, acupuncture should certainly be used to restore the balance of the body so that the problem does not return.

10.6 Pinguecula

Pinguecula are small translucent lumps on the sclera and conjunctiva. They are usually found on the medial side, on the same level as the center of the pupil. They may be on the sclera, or they may creep onto the surface of the cornea. It is unusual for them to go so far into the cornea as to cause any visual disturbance. In the early stage, the main reason that a patient would come for treatment is anxiety concerning the condition. At later stages, the patient may experience discomfort or even pain. Pain occurs because the raised lump prevents the eyelid from moving smoothly over the eyeball.

TCM approach

To understand the treatment approach in TCM, it is helpful to remember that the sclera and conjunctiva are external mucous membranes, sharing some of the characteristics of the lung (being a mucous membrane) and some of the characteristics of the skin (being external). In this case, its kinship with the skin provides the key to its treatment, for pinguecula can be treated in much the same way as a lipoma. It would therefore be characterized in TCM as a deposit of phlegm.

Deposits like this take time to build up and arise from a body condition that allows for deposits of phlegm. Even this body condition takes time to build up. Therefore, the relatively innocuous symptom takes a long time to develop in much the same way that bony deposits in arthritis take a long time to build up.

Treatment

The condition is a chronic one and requires a long time to clear. A careful diagnosis must be made for each patient, bearing in mind that the root cause of the pinguecula is a deposition of phlegm. Rather than detailed treatment regimens, the principles of treatment are given here:

- Bring qi to the eyes.
- Tonify the overall qi.
- Clear phlegm from the system.

Advice on lifestyle is important. In particular, the patients should avoid phlegm-producing foods. Some patients benefit from avoiding gluten.

Western medical and acupuncture treatment

The Western treatment is surgery, and that is often the treatment of choice. This minor condition is a manifestation of a deep imbalance that has taken years to develop. Treatment by natural means, whether acupuncture or herbs, will be slow, and many patients may feel that it is not worth the time and effort for such a relatively small gain. The author has seen many patients with pinguecula when it accompanied other conditions. In these patients, treatment with acupuncture significantly improved the pinguecula, as the other conditions improved.

10.7   Blepharitis

Blepharitis is an irritation of the margin of the eyelid, often with flaking skin. There is intermittent burning discomfort and itching. The irritation may spread to the conjunctiva, making it red locally. Occasionally, there is secondary infection with purulent discharge.

TCM approach

Etiology and pathology

The etiology in Western medicine is not well understood. In Chinese medicine it is considered to be a result of damp-heat invading the Spleen and Liver, which then rises up to the eyes. Here it combines with wind to generate pain, redness, and discharge, all of which would be expected from the combination of wind and damp-heat. The damp-heat may originate from greasy or spicy foods, alcohol, and, in the case of Western patients, gluten intolerance. In addition to the eye symptoms, there may be many signs and symptoms of damp-heat and of thick phlegm, including:

- face may be pale or red
- skin is shiny in parts and flaky in others
- feeling of heaviness
- abdominal aches
- loose, bad-smelling stools
- slippery or soggy pulse
- tongue has either a thick or shiny coating; stringy saliva may also be present

Additional symptoms indicating gluten intolerance include:

- discharges of thick green mucus
- irregular stools

TREATMENT

TREATMENT PRINCIPLE: Bring qi to the eyes, clear damp-heat, and, if present, clear the thick phlegm.

Points that bring qi to the eyes include:

BL-1 *(jing ming)*
ST-2 *(si bai)*
GB-20 *(feng chi)*
M-HN-9 *(tai yang)*
GV-23 *(shen shu)*
LI-4 *(he gu)*

METHOD: Use the tonifying method for the local points. The near and distal points are needled with the moving method to direct qi to the eyes.

Points to clear damp-heat and thick phlegm include:

LR-8 *(qu quan)*
SP-6 *(san yin jiao)*
BL-18 *(gan shu)*
BL-20 *(pi shu)*

METHOD: The even or moving technique is used at all the points.

Advice

All food items likely to produce damp-heat should be avoided. These include the ones normally mentioned in the Chinese texts: spicy, greasy foods and alcohol. Many Western patients improve dramatically on excluding wheat and other gluten-containing foods from their diet.

Western medical and acupuncture treatment

There is no treatment to cure this condition, only measures to control the inflammation, pain, and, when appropriate, infection. Steroids are commonly used for treating the pain and irritation, and antibiotics are used for treating the bacterial infection.

I have experience in treating only a few cases of blepharitis, but I have spoken to many practitioners who have more experience. They confirm that the combination of acupuncture and excluding gluten from the diet is very effective in curing this condition.

Endnotes

1. The equivalent pattern for babies and toddlers is slightly different and is given a special category in Chinese medicine: Liver malnutrition rising to the eyes. In Western children it is rare to see malnutrition. However, it is common to see the precursor to this, the 'accumulation disorder,' which is near to the adult pattern of retention of food and is described in more detail in *Acupuncture in the Treatment of Children* (3rd ed., p. 26).

2. In a significant number of cases the inflammation is a result of a Herpes simplex viral infection. In such cases, the condition will not go away easily. A test can confirm the presence of the virus, but at present, there is no effective treatment for the viral infection. The test will merely put a name on the persistent infection.

3. This section is a modification of material that first appeared in *Acupuncture in the Treatment of Children* (3rd ed., p. 327).

4. This pattern is often seen in red-heads and in the smoldering heat of adolescence.

5. There is a 'mismatch' here. The pulse is often weak even though the patient does not show the signs and symptoms of qi deficiency.

6. Here we use the common names of corneal ulcer and corneal opacity, rather than the technical names of ulcerative keratitis and nebulae, respectively.

Chapter 11

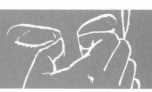

Problems of the Extraocular Muscles

11.1   Crossed Eyes in Children[1]

Crossed eyes[2] is the inability of one eye to attain binocular vision with the other eye because of an imbalance in usually one muscle of the affected eyeball. This symptom generally starts during childhood. If the symptom is treated soon after it is noticed or, at any rate, before the age of 14 years, there is a good chance of reversing the condition. If the symptom appears in a child younger than 8 years, the condition should be treated at once to prevent the weaker eye from going blind.[3]

Just as few people realize that acupuncture and other approaches can be used to treat near sightedness (Chapter 9), so also few people realize that acupuncture can be used for treating crossed eyes. It is often thought that surgery is the only option; but often acupuncture treatment can cure the condition. Moreover, the effect of acupuncture is to strengthen the eyes and so produce a long-lasting cure. Surgery, by contrast, weakens the eyes to a certain extent. Worse still, it is sometimes found that if convergent crossed eyes are corrected surgically during childhood, then divergent crossed eyes may develop as the body changes in adulthood.

Etiology

Western anatomy is helpful in providing an understanding of crossed eyes as it provides an insight into the mechanics of eye movement. We can then look to see how the functioning of the mechanical system of the eye is affected by the body's condition.

The eye is moved by three pairs of muscles (Fig. 11.1). The two that concern us are the horizontal ones. These muscles can only contract, and to move the eye left or right, only one of the muscles is needed. When the eye is at rest, all the muscles are relaxed, and the eye points forward. After moving the eye in a particular direction by contracting a muscle, relaxing that muscle allows the eye to spring back to its central position.

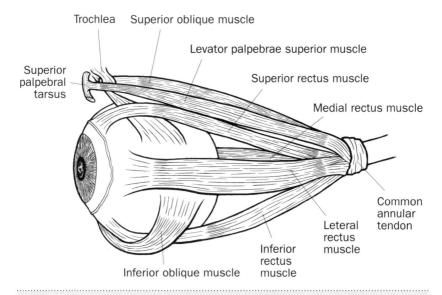

Fig. 11.1 Extraocular muscles

MECHANICAL DEFECTS

Shortened Muscle

In Western medicine, having crossed eyes is considered to be merely a mechanical defect: one of the muscles, usually the inward-pulling muscle, is too short. Surgical correction is seen as the only solution, with the shortened muscle being cut in a zigzag fashion to make it slightly longer.

Paralyzed Muscle

Another defect is paralysis of one of the eye muscles. When this happens, the eyes are parallel for much of the time because the movement is good in every direction except in the one relating to the paralyzed muscle. We will return to this below.

Diagnosis

For Caucasian children, this is usually quite easy. However, when diagnosing children of Oriental descent and young babies, it is easy to make a mistake because there is a fold of skin that makes it *look* as though the eye is not centrally located, even though it really is. The way to be sure is to take a pen-light and look for the reflection of this point of light in the child's lens. If the eyes are working well, the reflection will appear at exactly the same spot on the pupil of both eyes. If the eyes are crossed, the spot of light will appear in a slightly different position.

TCM approach

ETIOLOGY AND PATHOLOGY

Chinese medicine recognizes three main patterns that can lead to a shortened muscle. There are a total of four patterns if the pattern of paralyzed muscle is included. Each pattern has a slightly different cause:

- congenital
- hot lingering pathogenic factor
- overstimulation and overexcitement
- paralyzed eye muscle

Congenital

This simply means that the child is born with badly crossed eyes. It is quite common for children under 3 years of age to have slightly crossed eyes for it takes time to learn to use the eyes. Nonetheless, when a baby is relaxed, the eyes should be pointing in more or less the same direction.

Hot Lingering Pathogenic Factor

For some reason that is not clear, a hot lingering pathogenic factor can affect just one of the muscles unilaterally, and nearly always it is the one drawing the eye inward, shortening it. The muscle functions correctly, but since one muscle is shorter than the other, the eye is pulled inward, that is, the two eyes move together, both at the same time, but one is pulled inward. When such children arrive in the clinic, their eye movement is identical to that of children with congenital crossed eyes. The difference, however, is in their histories. In such cases, the children were born with straight eyes but acquired the symptom as a result of an infectious disease or an immunization.

Overstimulation and Overexcitement

On an energetic level, overstimulation and overexcitement corresponds to fire flaring up. It has a similar effect as a hot lingering pathogenic factor, the difference being that it is not a real fire. Rather, it is a false fire. The appearance of the eyes of a child with this condition is identical to that of the previous two patterns. Like the hot lingering pathogenic factor pattern, the child would have been born with normally working eyes and acquired the crossed eyes later on. The difference here is that there is no history of immunization or fever. Moreover, the child will appear overexcited, and the parents may notice that the eyes appear more or less crossed according to the child's level of tiredness or stimulation.

Paralyzed Eye Muscle

The etiology is the same as for a shortened muscle, only the effect is more severe: the fire blazing upward affects one or more of the channels around the eyes. In mild cases, when the fire subsides, a lingering pathogenic factor remains in the channels, causing shortening of the muscle. In extreme cases, the fire consumes the yin and leaves the muscle paralyzed. It is then a localized form of atrophy *(wei)* disorder. It is seen after a high fever, as in the Lung heat type of atrophy disorder, or after an immunization, especially the one for polio.

DIFFERENTIATING BETWEEN CROSSED EYES AND PARALYSIS OF AN EYE MUSCLE

The accompanying diagrams (Fig. 11.2) illustrate the difference in eye movements between a child who has straightforward crossed eyes as a result of a shortened muscle and a child who has paralysis of an eye muscle. It can be seen that the child who has a crossed eye can move both eyes together, but they never point in the same direction. It is similar to a motor car where the two front wheels have been set incorrectly. Both wheels change direction when the steering wheel is turned, but they are always at the same angle relative to each other and never parallel.

Crossed eyes:

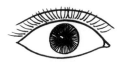 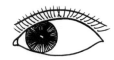

Looking to the right

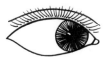 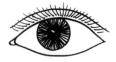

Looking ahead

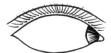 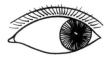

Looking to the left

Eyes are never parallel

Paralysis of muscle in the left eye:

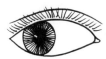 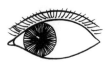

Looking to the right: eyes are parallel

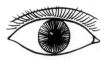 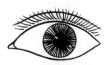

Looking ahead: eyes are parallel

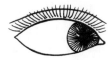 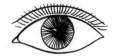

Looking to the left: left eye cannot move past the mid-point

Fig. 11.2 Sequence of diagrams showing the difference between crossed eyes and paralysis of an eye muscle

If a child has a paralyzed eye muscle, the movement is quite different. Looking one way, the eyes move perfectly together. Attempting to look the other way, one eye moves but the other eye gets 'stuck' just past the midpoint.

DIFFERENTIATION OF PATTERNS

Congenital

- born with crossed eyes

Hot Lingering Pathogenic Factor

- born with good eyes and then develops crossed eyes
- onset of the crossed eyes follows a fever or immunization
- swollen glands in the neck, under the ears, and/or in the groin
- some sign of redness on the face such as red cheeks or lips
- possible red tongue or red tip to the tongue
- irritable and restless

The latter four symptoms are typical of a lingering pathogenic factor pattern.

Overstimulation and Overexcitement

- born with good eyes and then develops crossed eyes
- eyes are more crossed when overtired or overexcited
- often has red cheeks
- lower back is often weak
- child is shy at first, then playful and overexcited
- tongue may be red or pale
- pulse rate varies with level of excitement

Paralyzed Eye Muscle

There are a large number of similarities between this pattern and the hot lingering pathogenic factor pattern for the simple reason that they are both the result of a fever. In this pattern, the fever has gone deeper and caused paralysis. Therefore, the same symptoms as listed above for a hot lingering pathogenic factor are often seen, with the only difference being in the movement of the eyes.

In some children the illness that caused the paralysis has left them with exhaustion and qi deficiency, rather than with a lingering pathogenic factor. In such cases, the following signs and symptoms will be seen:

- pale face
- tired, floppy demeanor
- poor appetite
- sleeps a great deal
- dull spirit in the eyes

TREATMENT

▶ *Congenital*

With the exception of 'womb heat' mentioned below, acupuncture is not all that effective. The child is born with a muscle that is too short. There are three ways that Western medicine can help:

1. As noted above, surgery to the affected muscle can be performed.
2. Strongly magnifying spectacles can be prescribed. This seems a strange thing to do, but it does appear to be effective. The reasoning behind it is as follows. When you try to focus the eyes on something close, they naturally tend to converge and cause the eyes to cross more. Putting strong spectacles on the child will tend to make the eyesight long-sighted, thereby creating a reflex action that will work in the opposite direction, causing divergence. This will help to correct the crossed eyes. This all assumes that the child has esotropia (convergent crossed eyes).
3. Orthoptic training, for example, eye exercises and patching the normal eye, can be given.

In some babies, the congenital crossed eyes are a result of womb heat, that is, heat that is present during the gestation. The signs and symptoms as well as the treatment are identical to that of a hot lingering pathogenic factor pattern. As one would expect of a problem present at birth, there is one small difference: it takes more treatments to be effective.

▶ *Hot Lingering Pathogenic Factor*

The main thrust of the treatment is to clear heat and benefit the eyes. Here is a prescription that I have found to be useful many times:

PC-7 (*da ling*)	Helps clear heat and is very beneficial in clearing this type of crossed eye pattern
LR-2 (*xing jian*)	In general, helps clear heat from the body and benefits the eyes, as it is a Liver channel point

This prescription is helpful when the main signs are those of heat, for example, insomnia or restlessness. If there are signs of the heat affecting another organ, for example, heat remaining in the Lungs causing recurrent cough, then this should also be treated with LU-7 *(lie que)* or LU-10 *(yu ji)*, for example. Additional points that can be of use include:

GB-1 *(tong zi liao)*	Useful for convergent crossed eyes
BL-1 *(jing ming)*	Useful for divergent crossed eyes
GB-20 *(feng chi)*	Brings qi to the eyes

NUMBER OF TREATMENTS: Treatment may be given up to three times a week, but even once a week can be effective. It is common to see a small improvement soon after the first treatment. Certainly, if there is no change after five treatments, then the treatment is not working. Typically, 10 to 15 treatments are enough.

▶ *Overstimulation and Overexcitement*

Acupuncture treatment of the presenting symptom of crossed eyes may or may not be effective. Children with this pattern are often prone to panic at the sight of the needle. If this occurs, then the appropriate treatment is to use the moxibustion stick on BL-23 and KI-1 with the aim of bringing down the qi and strengthening the water phase.

The most important part of the treatment is giving advice to the parents. It is absolutely essential that the child's level of stimulation be reduced. This may mean drastic measures, such as no television, avoiding playing with friends or relations who get them overexcited, or staying at home and pursuing quiet activities like drawing rather than going out for activity.

NUMBER OF TREATMENTS: It is always worth giving some tonifying treatments to strengthen the water phase and calm down overexcitement. It is also worthwhile arranging several appointments (say, five) so that the child's progress can be monitored and support provided to the parents in their attempts at reducing the level of the child's stimulation. Advice given at the first appointment without several follow-up visits is unlikely to be acted upon.

▶ *Paralyzed Eye Muscle*

The main treatment is to bring qi to the eyes and, in particular, to the affected muscle. The points that are used are similar to those used in the treatment of near sightedness:

GB-20 *(feng chi)*	Brings qi to the eyes
LI-4 *(he gu)*	Brings qi to the eyes
PC-6 *(nei guan)*	Brings qi to the eyes

Additionally, a point that is near the eye and nearest to the affected muscle is used, for example, one of the following:

GB-1 *(tong zi liao)*	Brings qi to an eye that will not move outward
BL-1 *(jing ming)*	Brings qi to an eye that will not move inward

NUMBER OF TREATMENTS: Since this pattern is a form of atrophy disorder *(wei syndrome)*, many treatments are required. They are best given as soon as possible after the onset of paralysis. Just as in treating paralysis after a stroke, treatment is very effective if started within three months of the paralysis. If two years have elapsed since onset, there may still be good results. More likely, however, very little at all will change as a result of the treatment.

Treatment ideally should be given every day for 10 days, followed by a 5-day rest before resuming treatment (one course of treatment). Five to 10 such courses may be required, a large number of treatments and an amount that few parents are prepared to undertake regardless of the cost. However, acupuncture is one of the very few treatments that has a chance of curing paralysis in an eye muscle.

If the patient is unable to come every day for 10 days, or even every weekday for two weeks, it is still worth treating *if the patient comes three times a week*. If they can only manage to come once or twice a week, it is generally not worth planning a long course of treatment. It is still worth giving a few treatments, however, as this will bring qi to the eyes, which may produce a miracle. A possible alternative to frequent acupuncture treatment is the frequent use of microcurrent electrical stimulation (see Section 6.2).

AUTHOR'S EXPERIENCE

The author has treated many children with crossed eyes.

General advice

- All patterns of crossed eyes can benefit from the series of eye massages presented in Section 6.2.

- It can be helpful to put a patch over the good eye to encourage the use of the lazy eye. However, it is quite difficult to get children to do this for any length of time. Strangely, it is sometimes just as effective putting the patch over the lazy eye. This seems to encourage the flow of qi to both eyes. It also accords with the old acupuncture principle of treating the good side to benefit the bad.

Endnotes

1. This chapter is a modified version of a chapter that first appeared in *Acupuncture in the Treatment of Children* (3rd ed., 1999).

2. Crossed eyes, also known as 'squint,' is part of the family of conditions grouped under the technical name of strabismus. Strabismus includes the paralytic condition as well as the nonparalytic conditions. The latter includes conditions where the deviation converges (esotropia), diverges (exotropia), or occurs in the vertical plane (hyper- or hypotropia).

3. Reduced visual acuity (amblyopia) results from suppression by the nervous system of the image from the deviating eye to avoid the confusion of double sightedness (diplopia). It is interesting to note that the converse may occur, that is, if an eye is not used, say, because of a disease, then strabismus can set in.

Chapter 12

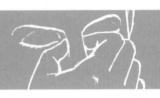

Miscellaneous Problems

12.1 Recovery after Eye Surgery

TCM approach

Surgery is frequently used on the eye to treat, for example, cataracts, corneal implants, adjustment of the lens in near sightedness, and retinal detachment. Frequently, patients come to us having made up their mind that they are going to have surgery and nothing will deter them from their course. However, we have something to offer these patients: we can bring qi to their eyes!

From the point of view of Chinese medicine, an eye disease cannot occur when the qi in the eyes is flowing well. It is also true that the eyes need qi in order to heal after surgery. It follows that a diseased eye will only heal slowly unless something is done to encourage the flow of qi.

TREATMENT

In my experience, very simple points—the basic points for bringing qi to the eyes—can be of use, including the following:

BL-2 *(zan zhu)*   LI-4 *(he gu)*

M-HN-8 *(qiu hou)*   GB-37 *(guang ming)*

GB-20 *(feng chi)*

Using these points can make a great difference in the rate of recovery, maybe even the difference between a successful operation and one that fails.

METHOD: The points should be tonified two to three times during the two weeks prior to the operation, with the last treatment being within a few days of the operation. Treatment should resume as soon as possible after the operation, preferably the next day.

FREQUENCY: The number of treatments that are given after an operation should be adjusted for each patient. Some patients experience a lot of pain either before or after surgery. In these cases, it is worth giving treatment every day. Yet for other patients, the treatment given before the operation is enough, and it is not necessary to give any treatment at all after the surgery.

RESULTS: The benefits of treatment are twofold. First, the pain normally experienced after an operation is much less, and second, the healing is accelerated. In the absence of controlled trials, one can only go on one's impressions. I believe that the time taken to heal is reduced to one-half or even one-third the expected time.

A small trial of the effect of a single acupuncture treatment on postoperative eye pain was published in *Abstracts of Clinical Experience with Acupuncture* (p. 313). The study used a combination of local, near, and distal points, depending on the location and nature of the pain. Of 19 patients, 11 were much improved, six had some improvement, and one had no change.

Author's experience

The author has treated many patients before surgery on various parts of the body, and a handful of patients before and after eye surgery. The improvement noted in eye patients was similar to that noted in other patients. Therefore, I think it is reasonable to assume that the improvement in recovery that is seen in general surgery applies equally to eye surgery.

Homeopathy

Homeopathic Arnica is also very helpful in treating the trauma of surgery. It is more general in its effect than acupuncture, and both may be given to good effect.

12.2   Seasonal Affective Disorder (SADS)

SADS is characterized by depression that is worse in the dark months of the year. It is quite natural for people to feel a bit depressed in winter spent in high latitudes, but this condition is much more pronounced than just gloom. It is serious depression! Moreover, it is strongly related to light levels. In severe cases, depression sets in soon after the autumnal equinox and does not lift until the spring equinox. It can be helped somewhat by daily exposure to high intensity full-spectrum lighting. Thus, it is very different from a weather-related depression, which typically may start in November or December and continue well into March or April when the weather starts to improve.

The condition has only been recognized fairly recently, so relatively little has been written about it and even less concerning effective treatments. I have not found anything about it in the Chinese texts, so inevitably what I write here is based entirely on my own experience and on other sources.

Anthroposophical medical perspective

In turning elsewhere for guidance, I have looked in particular to Anthroposophical medicine, a system developed by the visionary Rudolph Steiner.[1] He introduced the idea of a 'light metabolism.' He postulated that people need a certain amount of light in order to remain healthy, just as they need a certain amount of vitamins. If, for one reason or another, they do not obtain this light, then they will not feel well. In his writings, Steiner does not specifically address SADS, but he does notice that definite physiological changes take place in those who become blind.

TCM approach

ETIOLOGY AND PATHOLOGY

Based on Dr. Steiner's ideas, SADS is considered to be a result of faulty light metabolism. It would appear to be based on experience and the basic theory that there are two underlying causes: Liver weakness and Spleen weakness. Either the Liver is not absorbing the light (by means of the visual purple) or the Spleen is not transporting the light to where it is needed. These factors lead me to postulate the following patterns, which I have indeed seen in clinical practice:

- Liver blood insufficiency
- Liver and Kidney weakness
- Spleen and Heart yang deficiency

In addition to these energetic imbalances, there is a strong mental component. The patients have a basic underlying depression, which is there all the time. Even at the midsummer solstice, they are not usually brimming over with joy. When it comes to clinical practice, it is much easier to treat the seasonal aggravations than to cure the often deeply buried depression.

PATTERNS

▶ *Liver Blood Insufficiency*

The physical causes include heavy menstruation, loss of blood during childbirth, loss of blood through an accident, or an unbalanced vegetarian diet (see Appendix 2). Commonly, this pattern affects mothers who have the sole care of young children and who are exhausted through lack of sleep and lack of privacy. Signs and symptoms include:

- pale, gray face
- palpitations
- may live off nervous energy
- pale tongue
- choppy pulse

▶ *Liver and Kidney Weakness*

The Liver and Kidneys gradually weaken as one ages. There may also be a more rapid reduction in the Liver and Kidneys at menopause. Other factors can include burnout from overwork, any period of prolonged stress, or living in unhappy circumstances. Signs and symptoms:

- overall exhaustion
- weak back and knees
- difficulty concentrating
- may feel cold
- weak pulse

▶ *Spleen and Heart Yang Deficiency*

The common cause is poor diet and irregular eating habits combined with a sedentary lifestyle. These factors may be compounded by long hours of mental work. Signs and symptoms include:

- poor digestion
- bloating
- tendency to become overweight
- slippery or soggy pulse

TREATMENT

The points given below are for illustrative purposes only. In clinical practice, the prescription should be tailored to the individual and the time of year. It should also be borne in mind that it is well worth treating during the summer months, in preparation for the winter.

▶ *Main Points*

LR-3 *(tai chong)*
PC-7 *(da ling)*
PC-8 *(lao gong)*

METHOD: The even or tonifying method is used at LR-3 *(tai chong)*, possibly with moxibustion on the needle. The even method is used at PC-7 *(da ling)*, and moxibustion is to be performed at PC-8 *(lao gong)*.

▶ *Liver Blood Insufficiency*

TREATMENT PRINCIPLE: tonify the Liver blood.

LR-8 *(qu quan)*	Tonifies the Liver blood
BL-18 *(gan shu)*	Tonifies the Liver

METHOD: Use the tonifying method at all the points, with moxibustion on the needle. Also see Appendix 2.

▶ *Liver and Kidney Weakness*

TREATMENT PRINCIPLE: Tonify and strengthen the Liver and Kidneys.

BL-18 *(gan shu)*	Strengthens the Liver and Kidneys
BL-23 *(shen shu)*	Strengthens the Liver and Kidneys
CV-4 *(guan yuan)*	Strengthens the Kidneys
KI-7 *(fu liu)*	Tonifies the Kidney yang

METHOD: The method is used at all the points. Moxibustion may be used after needling.

▶ *Spleen and Heart Yang Deficiency*

TREATMENT PRINCIPLE: Tonify the Spleen and Heart yang.

ST-36 (*zu san li*)	Tonifies the Stomach and Spleen
SP-6 (*san yin jiao*)	Tonifies the Spleen
HT-7 (*shen men*)	Tonifies the Heart

In addition, add either

BL-15 (*xin shu*)	Strengthens the Heart
BL-20 (*pi shu*)	Strengthens the Spleen

or

CV-17 (*shan zhong*)	Brings qi to the Heart
CV-12 (*zhong wan*)	Front alarm point of the Spleen

METHOD: The tonifying method is used at all the points. Alternatively, simply use moxibustion.

RESULTS

If there is a clear energetic imbalance, with signs and symptoms matching a pattern, then the results will be good. When the patient does not show a special energetic imbalance, it means that the problem is more on the psychological level; as a consequence, it may be harder to treat.

If, during the course of treatment the patient either takes on a new occupation or manages to see their occupation in a more favorable light, the prognosis is good. If not, then it is unlikely that a complete cure will take place, and the treatment is then supportive during the winter months.

12.3 After-effects of a Stroke

A stroke, or cerebrovascular accident, can injure the eyesight. The injury may be in the part of the brain that perceives light, or it may be nearer to the eye itself. There is a characteristic pattern to the blindness, which varies depending on the site of the injury. However, for the purposes of treatment, it is not necessary to know the exact location of the injury. The important thing is to get on and give treatment—as soon as possible and lots of it! If the treatment is given straightaway after the stroke, and provided that the stroke is not too great, the patient has a chance of recovering the eyesight completely.

TCM approach

The following rules apply to stroke rehabilitation, regardless of whether the main loss of sensation and movement is in the eye or elsewhere in the body.

- *Intensive treatment must be given.* The ideal is once a day for 10 days, with a 4-day rest, but once a day for 5 days with a 2-day rest is a good second best. If the patient has only one treatment a week, it is unlikely that there will be much improvement. An alternative to daily treatment is the home use of a microcurrent electrical stimulator (see Section 6.2).

- *This intensity of treatment should be continued for about 100 treatments.* To many acupuncturists this may seem like a large number of treatments, but if it holds out the hope of restoring eyesight, it is well worth it. Some patients may balk at the cost, but it should be pointed out that the cost of such a course of treatment is likely to be less than a week's stay in a hospital bed.

- *Treatment is much more effective if it is started within 3 months of the nerve injury.* If it is started more than 2 years after the injury, it is likely that only minor changes will take place.

TREATMENT

Frequent local stimulation, preferably reaching the optic nerve, is the number-one aim of treatment. The details of the treatment may be left to the practitioner. Here we give a typical prescription of points that may be used with conventional acupuncture. The points around the eye may also be chosen for stimulation with a personal microcurrent electrical stimulator.

▶ *Typical Prescription*

BL-1 (*jing ming*)	Brings qi to the eyes
M-HN-8 (*qiu hou*)	Brings qi to the eyes

⌄

GB-20 (feng chi)	Brings qi to the eyes
ST-36 (zu san li)	Tonifies the overall qi
LR-3 (tai chong)	Regulates the Liver and benefits the eyes

Alternatives to ST-36 and LR-3 include:

BL-18 (gan shu)	Strengthens the Kidneys and Liver
BL-20 (pi shu)	Strengthens the Spleen and Liver
BL-23 (shen shu)	Strengthens the Kidneys and Liver

METHOD: When needling local points such as BL-1 *(jing ming)*, ST-1 *(cheng qi)*, and M-HN-8 *(qiu hou)*, the sensation should reach the back of the eye. Ideally, this should be a warm, comfortable sensation. In the later stages of treatment, when the qi is flowing well, these points need only be needled to a depth of 0.5 unit to get the sensation going immediately to the back of the eye. However, in the early stages of treatment, it may be necessary to needle to a heroic depth of 2 units before any sensation is felt at the back of the eye. (See Chapter 5 for further notes on needling these sensitive points.)

When needling near points, such as GB-20 *(feng chi)*, again the ideal is to get the sensation going to the eye, but treatments can often be effective in patients where you only manage to get local qi sensation. The distal points ST-36 *(zu san li)*, LR-3 *(tai chong)*, BL-18 *(gan shu)*, BL-20 *(pi shu)*, and BL-23 *(shen shu)* are needled with the tonifying method.

RESULTS: If the treatment rules given above are followed, there is a good chance that daylight eyesight will be completely restored. There may still be some slight reduction of nighttime vision in the affected areas.

AUTHOR'S EXPERIENCE

The author has treated many patients in China, and a few in the West, for the after-effects of stroke. Only one of these had serious loss of vision. However, the changes were so great in this patient that I nevertheless felt confident in presenting this chapter.

Microcurrent electrical stimulation

The microcurrent stimulator is of great benefit in treating the after effects of stroke since the patient or the patient's relatives can do the treatments up to three times a day without the need for coming to the clinic. With this frequency of treatment, the patient need only come to the clinic once or twice a week to regulate the overall qi.

12.4   Stye

TCM approach

Stye is the common word for a hordeolum, a swelling and (usually) inflammation of the hair follicle on the eyelids. From the point of view of Chinese medicine, the stye itself is categorized as wind-heat. The acupuncture treatment for wind-heat is very simple and is directed at the symptom.

According to *Essential Subtleties on the Silver Sea* (p. 204), the underlying pattern is heat toxin in the yang brightness *(yang ming)* channels as a result of indulging in excessive hot foods, spicy foods, and alcohol. Ingestion of excessive amounts of 'junk food,' that is, denatured foods containing large amounts of colorings and preservatives, can be added to this list.

Typically, patients who get styes tend to have red faces and greasy skin. They also tend to have the symptoms associated with heat toxin or damp-heat. Styes are more common in those under 40 years of age. The condition seems to be less common now.

TREATMENT

▶ *Wind-Heat*

TREATMENT PRINCIPLE: clear wind-heat and move local stagnation.
A frequently used prescription is the following:

LI-4 *(he gu)*	Clears wind
M-HN-6 *(yu yao)* or ST-2 *(si bai)*	Local points

METHOD: LI-4 *(he gu)* is needled bilaterally. M-HN-6 *(yu yao)* is needled on the affected side for a stye on the upper eyelid, and ST-2 *(si bai)* is needled on the affected side for a stye on the lower eyelid. Use the dispersing method at all the points. Treatment is given daily, and usually three or four treatments are enough. In very severe cases, prick the stye with a three-edged needle so that a few drops of blood come out.

▶ *Underlying Pattern*

Points that are useful for the underlying condition include the following:

SP-9 (*yin ling quan*)	Clears damp-heat
LR-13 (*zhang men*)	Clears stagnation in the middle burner and clears damp-heat
ST-44 (*nei ting*)	Clears heat from the Stomach channel (and so prevents heat from entering the eyelids)

METHOD: An even or dispersing method is used at all the points.

12.5   Entropion (Inverted Eyelids)

Entropion is only a small misalignment of the extremity of the eyelid, but the consequences of this minute structural change can be devastating for the sight because the inversion means that the eyelashes also turn inward, scratching the conjunctiva every time the eyelids are moved. The scratching is painful and quickly leads to inflammation. The normal treatment in Western medicine is minor surgery to shorten the exterior surface of the eyelid so that the eyelashes are pulled out of the eye and serve their proper purpose. This treatment can be effective, but there is the huge disadvantage that once the eyelids have started to change in this way, they become unstable. As a result, another operation may be needed a year or so later, either to further shorten the exterior surface or, occasionally, to undo the work of the first operation in cases where the patient's condition has improved.

TCM approach

Chinese medicine offers an alternative to surgery and the possibility of a long-term cure. The condition is described in *Essential Subtleties on the Silver Sea* (p. 236) as being due to an imbalance where there is both Lung heat and Spleen dampness. The reasoning is easy to understand. The exterior surface of the eyelid is governed by the Spleen. When dampness accumulates, the exterior surface becomes swollen. The interior surface of the eyelid is an extension of the conjunctiva and as such is governed by the Lungs. When heat affects the Lungs, the inner surface tends to contract. Thus, the exterior swelling and the interior contraction lead to the eyelid turning inwards.

Essential Subtleties on the Silver Sea describes a complicated procedure involving clamping and moxibustion on the eyelid itself. This must be learned from someone experienced in the technique. For those who do not have this opportunity, there is nevertheless much that can be done. Merely by bringing qi to the eyes, some relief will be obtained. By providing further treatment for the underlying condition, there is a possibility of curing the condition.

Pattern	Signs and Symptoms
Lung heat	Red face with white forehead History of Lung problems Possible asthma Rapid pulse, full in the Lung position
Spleen dampness	Gray face Eyelids slightly swollen or puffy Possible allergies to food Bloating Tendency to become overweight Slippery or soft pulse

TREATMENT

▶ *Main points*

To bring qi to the eyes and eyelids, use points such as:

ST-2 *(si bai)*
M-HN-6 *(yu yao)*
TB-23 *(si zhu kong)*

▶ *Lung Heat*

TREATMENT PRINCIPLE: Clear Lung heat.

LU-10 *(yu ji)*
LI-4 *(he gu)*

▶ *Spleen Dampness*

TREATMENT PRINCIPLE: Drain Spleen dampness.

ST-44 *(nei ting)*
SP-9 *(yin ling quan)*
CV-12 *(zhong wan)*

Note: The points listed here are of course just a place to start. In practice, the eye problem may be related to a deeper and long-lasting condition such as over-weight (in the case of Spleen dampness) or asthma (in the case of Lung heat). The treatment of these conditions requires more than just a few treatments with a few points. However, any trained acupuncturist will be familiar with the treatment of such conditions.

AUTHOR'S EXPERIENCE

The author has not had the opportunity to treat patients with this condition. However, I have observed the relationship between Lung heat and Spleen dampness in some acquaintances.

Endnotes

1. Dr. Steiner had little or no contact with Oriental ideas and almost certainly had no contact with Chinese medicine. However, working from first principles, he derived a system of medicine that has startling similarities to Chinese medicine. It is couched in the terminology of the Theosophical movement, which makes it very difficult for the uninitiated to understand. However, once the basic ideas have been grasped, the importance of his work can be understood. What is especially interesting is the ability of this system to bridge the gap between the large scale description of the human body in terms of the five phases (or the four elements, in his case) and the molecular structure of important compounds in the body.

Bibliography

Academy of Traditional Chinese Medicine. *Simplified Edition of Acupuncture (Zhen jiu xue jian bian)*. Beijing: People's Health Publishing Company, 1978.

Benjamin, H. *Better Sight Without Glasses*. London: Harper Collins, 1992.

Chengdu College of Traditional Chinese Medicine. *Acupuncture (Zhen jiu xue)*. Chengdu: Sichuan People's Press, 1981.

Coakes, R. and P. H. Sellors. *Outline of Ophthalmology*. Oxford: Butterworth Heinemann, 1995.

Sun Ssu-Miao. *Essential Subtleties on the Silver Sea (Yin hai jing wei)*. Kovacs, J. and P. U. Unschuld (trans.) Berkeley: University of California Press, 1998.

Guangdong Institute of Chinese Medicine. *Glossary of Chinese Medicine (Zhong yi da ci dian)*. Chengdu: Sichuan People's Press, 1984.

Hollwich, F. *Pocket Atlas of Ophthalmology*. F. C. Blodi (trans.). Stuttgart, Germany: Thieme, 1981.

Hoy Ping Yee Chan. *Window of Health: Ocular Diagnosis and Periocular Acupuncture*. Seattle: Northwest Institute of Acupuncture and Oriental Medicine, 1996.

Jiao Guo-Rui (ed.) *Abstracts of Clinical Experience with Acupuncture (Zhen jiu lin chuang jing yan ji yao)*. Beijing: People's Health Publishing Company, 1981.

Li Wen-Rui and He Bao-Yi (eds.) *Practical Acupuncture (Shi yong zhen jiu xue)*. Beijing: People's Health Publishing Company, 1982.

Maciocia, G. *The Practice of Chinese Medicine*. Edinburgh: Churchill Livingstone, 1994.

Parr, J. *Introduction to Ophthalmology*. Oxford: Oxford University Press, 1978.

Shanghai College of Traditional Chinese Medicine. *Acupuncture: A Comprehensive Text (Zhen jiu xue)*. O'Connor, J. and D. Bensky (trans.) Chicago: Eastland Press, 1981.

Scott, J. and T. Barlow. *Acupuncture in the Treatment of Children* (3rd ed.) Seattle: Eastland Press, 1999.

Sun Xue-Quan (ed.) *Collection of Clinical Experiences with Acupuncture (Zhen jiu lin zheng ji yan)*. Jinan: Shandong Technical Press, 1982.

Tianjin College of Traditional Chinese Medicine, No. 1 Affiliated Hospital. *Practical Acupuncture (Shi yong zhen jiu xue)*. Tianjin: Tianjin Science and Technology Press, 1980.

Yan Hong-Chen and Cheng Shao-En (eds) *Anthology of Acupuncture Prescriptions (Zhen jiu chu fang ji)*. Guilin: Guilin People's Publishing Company, 1983.

Zhang Wang-Zhi. *Key Points of Ophthamology (Yǎn kē tàn lí)*.* Hunan: Hunan Technical Publishing House, 1982.

Eye and Throat Diseases in Traditional Chinese Medicine (Zhong yi yan hou ke xue). Chengdu: Sichuan People's Press, 1980.

---

* Although this is a book about ophthalmology, the literal translation of its title is *Leading Out a Black Horse*.

Appendix 1

Summary of Patterns

▶ Retinal Problems:

Optic atrophy, macular degeneration, retinitis pigmentosa, and night blindness	Liver and Kidney weakness
	Heart nourishment (*ying*) deficiency
	Spleen and Kidney yang deficiency
	Qi and blood stagnation
	Accumulation of phlegm
Optic neuritis and papilledema	Liver yang rising
	Heart and spirit injured
	Stomach heat

▶ Fluid Problems:

Glaucoma (acute closed-angle)	Liver yang rising
	Kidney weakness
	Heart panic
	Nervous excitability

⌄

Glaucoma (chronic open-angle)	Liver yang rising
	Kidney weakness
	Spleen qi deficiency
	Lung qi deficiency
Watering eyes	Wind-heat
	Liver qi stagnation
	Lingering pathogenic factor
	Lung and Spleen qi deficiency
	Heart fire
	Bladder channel damp-heat
	Blood insufficiency
	Liver and Kidney weakness
Blocked tear duct	Liver qi stagnation
	Heart fire
	Lingering pathogenic factor
	Bladder channel damp-heat
	Lung and Spleen qi deficiency
	Liver and Kidney weakness

▶ Lens Problems:

Cataracts	Liver and Kidney yin deficiency
	Lung dryness and Lung heat
Myopia	Spleen qi deficiency
	Lingering pathogenic factor

▶ Problems of the Front of the Eye:

Acute conjunctivitis	Wind-heat
	Uprising heat and dampness
Chronic conjunctivitis	Liver and Gallbladder heat
	Liver and Kidney weakness

Hay fever	Liver yang rising
	Liver and Gallbladder damp-heat
	Lingering pathogenic factor
	Lung and Spleen qi deficiency
	Lung and Kidney deficiency
Corneal ulcer, opacity, and erosion	Liver and Kidney weakness
	Liver and Gallbladder heat
	Wind-heat
	Lung yin deficiency
Pinguecula	Phlegm
Blepharitis	Phlegm
	Damp-heat

▶ Problems of the Extraocular muscles:

Crossed eyes in children	Congenital
	Hot lingering pathogenic factor
	Overstimulation and overexcitement
	Paralyzed eye muscle

▶ Miscellaneous Problems:

Seasonal Affective Disorder (SADS)	Liver blood insufficiency
	Liver and Kidney weakness
	Spleen and Heart yang deficiency
Stye	Wind-heat with heat toxin in the yang brightness (*yang ming*) channels
Entropion (inverted eyelids)	Lung heat
	Spleen Dampness

Appendix 2

Treatment of Blood Insufficiency and Anemia

It is a widely held view that acupuncture is an inappropriate therapy for treating the condition of blood insufficiency and its close relation, anemia. It is often said that only herbs can cure this condition. The reasoning behind this belief is that blood insufficiency is a condition where there is not enough of the physical substance that makes up blood. It is argued that only herbs contain the physical substance that is required to restore the balance. This is an attractive argument, but it does not match clinical experience. The reality is that the condition has a related qi deficiency and also a related emotional attitude. For many patients in the West, these are more important than the physical deficiency. This means that treatments such as acupuncture, which treat qi imbalance and emotional attitudes, are effective in treating blood insufficiency.

There are many different approaches to treatment that depend somewhat on the patient to be treated. Therefore, rather than provide an exhaustive discussion, we reproduce here a series of prescriptions given in *Practical Acupuncture* (p. 351).

Prescription #	Acupuncture points
1	BL-43 (*gao huang shu*) GB-20 (*feng chi*) ST-36 (*zu san li*)
2	BL-23 (*shen shu*) GV-14 (*da zhui*) N-HN-54 (*an mian*)
3	LI-4 *(he gu)* LI-11 (*qu chi*) GV-4 (*ming men*)
4	BL-17 (*ge shu*) BL-18 (*gan shu*) BL-19 (*dan shu*)
5	BL-19 (*dan shu*) GV-14 (*da zhui*) N-HN-54 (*an mian*)
6	BL-23 (*shen shu*) ST-36 (*zu san li*) ST-44 *(nei ting)*

METHOD: Use one prescription each day for 6 days, and then rest for 3 days.

Appendix 3

More about Mercury

As discussed in Chapter 4 and elsewhere in the book, mercury can be a major factor leading to eye disease. Mercury can leach out of imperfect amalgam fillings, slowly infiltrating the upper jaw as far as the eyes. The circulation of fluids and also of energy may be severely affected, with consequent eye problems. This appendix covers some further relevant information regarding detection and elimination of this toxin.

Detection of mercury

The primary means of detecting heavy metal is by analysis of the hair, urine, or blood by chromatography or mass spectrometry. Neither of these methods is entirely reliable, for what is measured is the amount of the metal found in the respective body parts, not in other parts of the body. In many cases, the accumulation of mercury has occurred over many years and the amount of mercury being taken into the body each day is very small. Most of it is stored in the body (particularly in the kidneys and the bones), so very little will be found in the blood. Moreover, the fundamental problem is that each day a little more is being absorbed than is being excreted. Consequently, only very little may be found in the hair and the urine. Thus, the problem is not that the tests themselves are inaccurate but that the body is hiding the mercury in inaccessible places.

If mercury is suspected, and if for some reason it is essential to prove that mercury is present, there is a way of making it show itself. This is by a so-called 'challenge' test where a small round of chelation[1] detoxification is started. This involves introducing a chemical called sodium 2,3-dimercaptopropane-1-sulphonate (or DMPS for short) into the blood stream, usually by injection. This substance combines ('chelates') with heavy metals, which are then excreted through the urine. The amount of chelated mercury collected in the urine over the next 24 hours provides a measure of how much mercury is present in the body. The shortcoming is that DMPS combines with all heavy metals so the test may give a false reading if other heavy metals are present.

TIMES WHEN MERCURY IS MORE OF A PROBLEM

When the amount of mercury absorbed is greater than the amount excreted, the excess is stored in various parts of the body, most notably the kidneys and bones. During early life, the individual's energy is good and the toxins thus stored do not often give any trouble. The problems arise later in life when the bones and kidneys are saturated. It is especially a problem for women at menopause. This is because, in later life and during menopause, the bone density reduces. As this occurs, the calcium—as well as the mercury—leaves the bones. The mercury then enters the bloodstream, giving rise to a multitude of symptoms.

THE MERCURY TYPE

Why is it that some people's health is ruined by mercury fillings, while others are unaffected? At the present time, it is hard to predict accurately who will be adversely affected, but there are two guidelines that may help the practitioner give informed advice. The first is that mercury is more likely to be absorbed in those who drive themselves continuously without leaving time for relaxation. The other is that there is a recognizable 'mercury type'. During the 19th century, homeopaths observed the changes in character that took place in those who were poisoned by mercury and noticed various character traits that were emphasized. A full description of these traits is beyond the scope of this book, and readers are referred to the many excellent books on classical homeopathy that are now available.

Mercury Detoxification

AMINO ACID THERAPY

In a healthy body, mercury is excreted mainly through the large intestine and kidneys. The body combines the mercury with glutathione (a tripeptide) and cysteine (an amino acid)[2] and voids the resulting products in the urine and stools. The big problem for someone who has large amounts of mercury in the system is that mercury actually collects in the kidneys, impairing their function and so preventing the excretion of mercury.

Cysteine is found in most proteins, especially those found in meat, and glutathione is found in meat as well. Therefore, a way to encourage the excretion of mercury is to eat more meat. For vegetarians and those accustomed to a low-protein diet, this is not a possibility; for them, the extra amino acids can be introduced in pill form. A typical prescription is as follows:

- one 50-mg glutathione pill taken once a day to begin with, increasing to three times a day
- one 500-mg cysteine pill taken with one 1500-mg pill of vitamin C; the vitamin C is initially taken once a day, increasing to three times a day

There is also an algae called 'chlorella' that encourages the expulsion of mercury.

Chelation Therapy

The most reliable method is the so-called chelation therapy. Here the chemical injected is a modification of DMPS called DMSA. However, patients undergoing this treatment do report very uncomfortable side effects. To put it mildly, they feel very ill! There are a number of reasons for this, one of them being that good minerals are simultaneously being leached out of the body. Another reason is that it requires a lot of energy to excrete so much mercury.

It does seem that patients who undergo a complete course of chelation therapy do eventually get rid of all their mercury. The biggest problem is that the treatment is very draining to the energy and can even injure the health. Many patients simply cannot face continuing with course of treatment.

Alternatives to Chelation

Chelation therapy has its origins in Western medicine, which ignores the fact that humans are living beings and that energy is part of their makeup. The same chelation procedure is given to all patients, irrespective of their physique. This runs counter to the theories of Chinese medicine, which looks primarily at the energy pattern of the patient and then at the cause of disease. In the case of chronic mercury poisoning, the energy pattern is invariably deficiency compounded with fluid imbalance and long-term buildup of phlegm. Exactly *where* the deficiency occurs and exactly *where* the phlegm builds up may vary from patient to patient. However, from the point of view of Chinese medicine, the very first part of treatment would be to build up the patient's energy. This can only be done if the patient is prepared to rest and to undergo a fairly long course of treatment. One of the biggest problems is that it is the nature of mercury-laden patients to have great difficulty in giving up their work. They find rest almost intolerable. However, if the patient is prepared to take the time, she can save herself a lot of physical suffering, for then the more gentle methods can be used.

There are also Western herbs that can help in the detoxification. Foremost among these is bayberry (*Myrica cerifera*). This is a warm Spleen tonic with a special effect in clearing dampness. Its effect on clearing the symptoms of mercury poisoning have been well established in the 19th century when mercury poisoning was very common. (At that time, mercury was freely given for many diseases. It was almost the only medicine used in the treatment of syphilis. The treatment consisted of giving mercury "until salivation.")

How Chinese Medicine Can Help

Chinese medicine can help in a number of ways. It can be used to support the patient while they are undergoing the suffering of chelation therapy. Alternatively, Chinese medicine can be used as the primary therapy. My experience has been that both acupuncture and herbal medicine can be used. If treatment is given on the basis of the differentiation of patterns, the energy of the patient is so much improved that the mercury starts to leave the body. We know from the work of naturopathic physicians that proteins are required for this process, but there is no need for special proteins to be injected. The protein available in a meat-based diet is usually sufficient.

Principles of Acupuncture Treatment   As mentioned above, treatment should be given on the basis of the differentiation of patterns. Frequently, mercury poisoning gives rise to Spleen and Kidney yang insufficiency. However, there are some patients where the signs and symptoms are entirely different. The diagnosis and treatment should be determined on the basis of the patient's needs.

NEED FOR REST

In addition to medical treatments, patients who wish to eliminate mercury from the body need to rest. Mercury poisoning is like any other illness in that it needs energy to get better. Energy is needed to excrete mercury. In clinical practice, the first stage of the treatment is to settle the energy of the patient and to help her understand that she needs to take some time to rest and recover her energy.

DENTAL WORK

In order for mercury detoxification to be successful, it is obvious that the source of mercury has to be removed. In many cases, this is the mercury in the fillings in the mouth. It is therefore essential that these be removed. This itself is not without its problems. Experience with a number of patients, the author included, is that there can be long after effects of replacing mercury fillings with those made of other materials. It seems that the very act of removing them stirs up the mercury that has collected in the upper and lower jaws. It is common to have jaw ache, gingivitis, severe sinusitis, and quite bad memory loss for the following 6 to 12 months. This is even the case when meticulous care has been taken to avoid absorbing or swallowing any mercury during the dental work.

Endnotes

1. Chelation is the entrapment of a metal positive ion inside a 'cage' of a larger molecule. The tenacity of the trap varies with the metal ion and the cage. Chelation can form the basis of tests as well as treatment.

2. It is cysteine, not cystine, that binds mercury.

Appendix 4

Some Commonly Used Medicines

The normal medicines in general use—antibiotics, steroids, adrenaline, antihistamines, and nonsteroidal anti-inflammatories—make their appearance in ophthalmology, often in the form of drops. There are two medicines which are of great interest to us, as shown in the following table.

Adrenaline and related sympathetics, e.g., phenylnephrine and atropine	These have the effect of dilating the pupil and are often dropped in the eye prior to an examination so that the pupil is nice and wide and the investigator can see into the eye more easily. There is a tendency for adrenaline to raise the blood pressure, and that, combined with the relaxation of the pupil, makes its use dangerous in patients with glaucoma.
Pilocarpine and related chemicals	These drugs have the reverse effect. They constrict the pupil and lower intraocular pressure. They are the main medication for treating glaucoma. Although not officially acknowledged, there is some evidence that taking pilocarpine regularly makes a heart attack more likely. Pilocarpine is also used to produce sweating in sweat chloride tests.

Point Index

Note: Page numbers followed by a "t" indicate that the citation appears in a table.

ST-2, 48, 124t, 154, 175t, 177

ST-8, 51

ST-36, 56, 75t, 76t, 77t, 95t, 96, 101t, 110t, 111t, 119, 120t, 125t, 137t, 144t, 172t, 174t, 186t

ST-40, 76t, 143t

ST-44, 44, 82t, 176t, 177, 186t

ST-45, 82t

.... **T**

TRIPLE BURNER CHANNEL

TB-2, 54

TB-3, 54, 109t, 132t, 133t

TB-5, 78t, 133t

TB-17, 52, 118t

TB-20, 52

TB-23, 48, 124t, 177

General Index

Heart yang deficiency, 28–29
Heat toxin, in stye, 175, 183
Heavy metals
    in etiology of eye diseases, 41–44, 79
    in retinal problems, 73
Herbal medicine
    in watering eyes due to blood loss, 112
    vs. acupuncture, 15, 185
Hidden emotions, 40
High blood pressure, 117
    and elevated intraocular pressure, 97
Homeopathy
    for trauma of surgery, 168
    in treatment of cataract, 115
    in treatment of mercury poisoning, 188
Hordeolum, 175–176
Hot lingering pathogenic factor
    in crossed eyes, 159–160, 162, 163–164
    in extraocular muscle problems, 183
Hot tears, 103

······ **I**

Inferior oblique muscle, 25, 158
Inferior rectus muscle, 158
Inner canthus, 21
Inner Classic (Nei jing), 27
Innervation, 24–25
Interior rectus muscle, 25
Internal fluids, 23–24
Intestinal worms, signs in eyeball, 36
Intraocular bleeding, role of blood stasis in, 29
Intraocular fluids, role of Spleen in, 30
Intraocular pressure
    causes of elevated, 97–98
    in glaucoma, 85
    measurement of, 86–87
Iris, 20, 21, 23
    in closed-angle glaucoma, 88
    muscles controlling, 89
Itchy eyes, 35

······ **J**

Joy, in etiology of eye diseases, 39

······ **K**

Kidney exhaustion, 91

Kidney qi insufficiency, in retinal diseases, 75
Kidney weakness, 97
    in closed-angle glaucoma, 89, 90t, 181
    in follow-up treatment of closed-angle
        glaucoma, 93t
    in open-angle glaucoma, 98–99, 101, 181
Kidney yang deficiency, in lead poisoning, 43
Kidney yin deficiency, in cataract, 116
Kidneys
    excretory dysfunction from mercury
        poisoning, 42, 188
    governance of opening and closing by, 32
    relationship to eyes, 31–32
    role in development of cataract, 117

······ **L**

Lachrymal ducts, 24
Large Intestine channel, 33
Lateral rectus muscle, 25, 158
Lazy eye, 166. *See also* Crossed eyes
Lead poisoning, effects on eyes, 42–43
Lens, 20, 21, 23
    anatomy of, 116
    progressive hardening of, 32
    role of Kidneys in, 32
Lens problems, 115
    cataract, 115–121
    myopia in children and teenagers, 21–126
    pattern differentiation for, 182
Levator palpebrae superior muscle, 25, 158
Life problems, 57
Light, role of Liver in perception of, 28
Light metabolism, 169
Lingering pathogenic factor
    and near sightedness, 123–124, 125
    and phlegm in blocked tear ducts, 113
    in blocked tear duct, 182
    in crossed eyes, 159–160
    in hay fever, 139, 140–141, 143, 182
    in near sightedness, 182
    in watering eyes, 103, 104, 106, 110, 182
Liver yang rising
    in optic neuritis and papilledema, 81t
Liver, relationship to eyes, 27, 28
Liver and Gallbladder heat
    in chronic conjunctivitis, 136–137
    in corneal problems, 148–149, 150–151,
        183
    in hay fever, 139, 140, 143–144, 182

Optic neuritis, 79
and multiple sclerosis, 82–83
clinical results, 82
etiology and symptoms, 79–80
patterns of, 181
TCM approach to, 80–82
Treatment of, 80–82
Organs
imbalances as etiological factors in eye
disease, 57
relationship to eyes, 27–33
treating imbalances in, 58
Outer canthus, 21
Oversensitivity to light, 43
Overstimulation
in etiology of crossed eyes, 160, 162, 164,
183
in etiology of eye diseases, 39
role of phosphorous poisoning in, 43
Overwork, and closed-angle glaucoma, 89

.... **P**

Pain, 35. *See also* Dull pain; Stabbing pain;
Strong pain
Panic, in etiology of eye diseases, 39
Papilledema
etiology and symptoms, 80
patterns of, 181
Paralyzed muscle, 159
in crossed eyes, 160, 162–163, 183
treatment of, 165
Partial cataract, 120
Penetrating vessel, 33
Perception, role of Heart in, 29
Peripheral vision
in macular degeneration, 71
loss in retinitis pigmentosa, 71
Phlegm
accumulation through mercury
poisoning, 41, 190
and development of open-angle
glaucoma, 99
in blepharitis, 153–154, 183
in blocked tear ducts, 113
in pinguecula, 152, 153, 182
in retinal problems, 181
signs and symptoms of, 74t
treatment in retinal problems, 76t

Phosphorus poisoning, effects on eyes, 43–44
Pinching and pressing massage, 61
Pinguecula, 152–153
pattern differentiation for, 183
Plum blossom needle, 59–60. *See also* Electric
plum blossom technique
Poor color perception, 36
Posterior chamber, 20, 23
Practical Acupuncture, 185
Presbyopia, role of Kidneys in, 32
Progressive blindness, in optic atrophy, 69

.... **Q**

Qi
bringing to eyes, 57–58, 77
maintaining in eyes after treatments, 126
reduced in eyes, 75
Qi and blood stagnation
in retinal problems, 181
signs and symptoms of, 73t
treatment in retinal problems, 76t
Qi sensation, with deep needling of eyes, 45–46

.... **R**

Rage
in etiology of eye diseases, 39
relationship to eyes, 28
Red eyeball color, 36
Red eyes, walnut shell spectacles for, 63–64
Refractive index, of aqueous humor, 20
Repressed anger, and closed-angle glaucoma,
89
Results of treatment, 17
Retina, 20
anatomy of, 22, 70
Kidney influence on, 31
Retinal damage, effect of phosphorous
poisoning on, 44
Retinal degeneration
blood stasis and, 29
deep needling in, 45
Retinal problems
and loss of vision, 69
and multiple sclerosis, 82–83
clinical results, 78
emotional causes of, 73–75
frequency of treatment for, 77–78

Bates method, 63
electric plum blossom technique, 59–60
eye massage, 60–61
massaging BL-1, 62
massaging GB-20, 62
massaging LI-4, 62–63
microcurrent electrical stimulation, 64–67
pinching and pressing BL-1, 61
traditional Chinese massage, 60
walnut shell spectacles, 63–64
Triple Burner channel, 33
Trochlea, 25
Tunnel vision, in retinitis pigmentosa, 71
Turbid fluids, in development of cataract, 117

······· **U**

Ultraviolet light, and free radicals, 116
Upper eyelid, 29
Uprising heat and dampness, in acute
conjunctivitis, 131, 132, 133–134, 182

······· **V**

Vegetable fats, and free radicals, 116
Vision, normal development of, 121–122
Vision loss, due to retinal problems, 69
Visual display units (VDUs), 90
in etiology of eye diseases, 37–38
Visual purple, 22, 25, 169
effect of carrots on, 40
Liver role in governing, 28
Vitamin A, 25
as remedy for night blindness, 72
Vitamin supplements, in retinal problems, 79
Vitreous humor, 20, 22, 23

······· **W**

Walnut shell spectacles, 63–64
Watering eyes
Bladder channel damp-heat in, 107, 111
blocked tear ducts and, 113
blood insufficiency in, 104–105, 107–108,
111–112
etiology and pathology of, 105–108

Heart fire and, 107, 111
lingering pathogenic factor and, 106, 110
Liver and Kidney weakness in, 108, 112
Liver qi stagnation in, 105–106, 109–110
Lung and Spleen qi deficiency in, 106–107,
110–111
patterns in, 103–104, 182
TCM approach to, 102
tears and yin organs in, 104
treatment of, 108–112
wind-heat and, 105, 109
Weak qi, and near sightedness, 123, 124
Welder's eyes, 38, 134
Western medical treatment
of acute conjunctivitis, 134
of blepharitis, 155
of chronic conjunctivitis, 137
of closed-angle glaucoma, 94
of corneal problems, 151–152
of hay fever, 145
of near sightedness, 122
of open-angle glaucoma, 102–103
of pinguecula, 153
Wind-heat
and conjunctivitis, 37
in acute conjunctivitis, 131, 133, 182
in corneal problems, 148, 149, 183
in stye, 183
in watering eyes, 103, 104, 105, 109, 182
Women's Precious Pill, 112
Worry, in etiology of eye diseases, 39

······· **Y**

Yang Heel vessel, 33
Yellow eyeball color, 36
Yin consumption, and development of
cataract in diabetes, 117
Yin deficiency, in phosphorous poisoning, 43
Yin Heel vessel, 33
Yin organs, relationships to eyes, 27–33

······· **Z**

Zonule, 23